Lung Sounds .

CONTRIBUTORS

Cynthia A. Cline, BS, RRT
Instructor, Department of Respiratory Therapy
School of Allied Health Professions
Loma Linda University
Loma Linda, California

Douglas D. Deming, MD
Assistant Professor
School of Medicine
Loma Linda University
Medical Director, Neonatal-Pediatric Respiratory Care
Loma Linda University Medical Center
Loma Linda, California

James R. Dexter, MD, FCCP
Associate Professor
School of Medicine
Loma Linda University
Chief, Pulmonary Section
Jerry L. Pettis Memorial Veterans Hospital
Loma Linda, California

Susanne C. Lareau, RN, MS
Pulmonary Clinical Nurse Specialist
Jerry L. Pettis Memorial Veterans Hospital
Assistant Clinical Professor of Nursing
School of Nursing
Loma Linda University
Loma Linda, California

David B. Martin, MD
Department of Family Practice
Kaiser Permanente Hospitals
Fontana, California

LUNG SOUNDS

A Practical Guide

Robert L. Wilkins, MA, RRT
Assistant Professor and Associate Chairman
Department of Respiratory Therapy
School of Allied Health Professions
Loma Linda University
Loma Linda, California

John E. Hodgkin, MD
Clinical Professor of Medicine
University of California, Davis
Medical Director
Center for Health Promotion and Rehabilitation
Medical Director, Respiratory Care and Pulmonary
    Rehabilitation
St. Helena Hospital and Health Center
St. Helena, California

Brad Lopez, MS, RRT
Instructor
Respiratory Care Program
Fresno City College
Fresno, California

The C. V. Mosby Company

St. Louis • Toronto • Washington, D.C.

Executive Editor: David T. Culverwell
Production Coordinator: Lisa G. Cunninghis
Manuscript Production Editor: A. Tony Meléndez

Composition: Electro-Graphics
              Baltimore, Maryland

Library of Congress Cataloging-in-Publication Data

Wilkins, Robert L.
  Lung sounds.

  Accompanied by an audio-tape.
  Includes index.
    1. Auscultation. 2. Lungs—Diseases—Diagnosis. 3. Lungs—Examination.
I. Hodgkin, John E. (John Elliott), 1939-   . II. Lopez, Brad. III. Title. [DNLM:
1. Auscultation—methods. 2. Lung. 3. Respiratory Sounds. WF 600 W685L]
RC734.A94W54   1988   616.2'407544   87-24748
ISBN 0-8016-5532-3

                9 8 7 6 5 4 3 2 1

Printed in the United States of America

CONTENTS

PREFACE

Chest auscultation represents an inexpensive and efficient way to evaluate lung function. It is often utilized only in a cursory manner since many clinicians rely so heavily on the chest x-ray, arterial blood gas and spirogram to evaluate the patient's pulmonary status. This superficial utilization of chest auscultation is often accompanied by a poor understanding of the mechanisms and clinical significance of lung sounds. Fortunately, recent research has supplied important insight into the understanding of lung sounds. With this in mind, we have written this text accompanied with an audio-tape to help clinicians better understand and apply lung sounds to patient care.

This text and audio-tape have been developed to teach students in nursing, respiratory therapy, physician assistants, and medical school programs about lung sounds. Any practicing clinician who auscultates patients should also find the text and audio-tape helpful as a review and update.

To help the beginning student, the text begins with a review of pulmonary anatomy and physiology, highlighting the points important for auscultation. Anatomy and physiology for the adult and neonate are presented in Chapter 1. This material, along with Chapter 2, is intended only to provide enough background information to clarify the remaining chapters.

Chapter 2 presents an overview of patient assessment. This chapter shows how auscultation "fits into" the total process of patient evaluation. It is not intended to teach chest diagnosis, but does briefly describe how patients with lung disease are evaluated. Most importantly, this chapter describes how to auscultate.

Chapter 3 reviews the terminology to utilize in describing lung sounds. This chapter also presents the current understanding of the mechanisms responsible for producing normal and abnormal lung sounds. This information is crucial to anyone trying to utilize chest auscultation as an assessment tool.

Chapter 4 describes the clinical application of lung sounds. The latest research describing the clinical significance of lung sounds can be found here. This chapter will help clinicians learn how to interpret the auscultatory findings.

Chapter 5 is a presentation of seven case examples illustrating how auscultatory findings can be very useful in evaluating patients with pulmonary disease. For the novice, Chapter 5 should be read only after Chapters 1–4 have been studied and after the adult and neonatal lung sound examples on the audio-tape have been mastered. To make the case samples of Chapter 5 more realistic, we have provided the auscultatory findings specific to each case in the final section of the audio-tape.

A list of the lung sound examples recorded on the tape is provided at the conclusion of the text in the appendix. The audio-tape is most realistically listened to by use of a stethoscope with the volume set relatively low. The diaphragm of the stethoscope should be placed 2–3 inches from the speaker of the cassette player.

The authors are grateful to numerous individuals for assistance in the completion of this project. We appreciate the typing done by Linda Dortch and the editorial assistance of Ruby Wilkins. Don Cicchetti's expertise was instrumental in preparing the audio-tape.

DEDICATION

To our spouses and children

Robert L. Wilkins	Kristi, Tyler and Nicholas
John E. Hodgkin	Jeanie, Steven, Kathryn, Carolyn, Jonathan and Jamie
Brad Lopez	Jan, Ted and Justin

CHAPTER
1
Pulmonary Anatomy and Physiology

OBJECTIVES

After reading this chapter, the learner should be able to recognize and describe:

1. Pulmonary anatomy and physiology structures in the adult and infant.

2. Pulmonary mechanics and intrathoracic forces that occur during breathing.

3. Normal lung volumes and capacities in the adult.

4. The topographical position of lung borders and fissures.

5. The mechanical properties of the chest wall and lung in the neonate.

The major purpose of the lung is gas exchange. On inspiration, atmospheric air enters the airways and travels to the alveoli. Oxygen diffuses from the alveolus through the alveolar-capillary membrane into the blood, and carbon dioxide diffuses from the blood into the alveolus. This is known as respiration. During exhalation, gas moves from the alveoli toward the upper airways and is exhaled through the mouth and nose into the atmosphere. The exchange of air between the lungs and the atmosphere is known as ventilation. This continuous process of ventilation and respiration depends on a patent airway system, intact pulmonary parenchyma, adequate blood flow to the lung and a normal neuromuscular system.

Pulmonary Anatomy

Airways

During spontaneous breathing, air enters the upper airways which consist of the oral and nasal cavities, pharynx, and larynx (see Fig. 1-1). The primary function of the upper airways is to prepare the inspired air for entry into the lungs. The nasal passages are particularly designed to act as an "air conditioner." The nasal turbinates and mucous membranes in the nasal cavity warm, filter, and humidify the inspired air during inspiration. Filtering of the inspired air is accomplished in part by the strong hairs of each nostril. A rich network of blood vessels in the mucosal membrane is instrumental in warming and humidifying the inspired air. While the entire respiratory tract can serve to warm and moisten the inspired air, the nose normally provides the greatest percentage of this function.

Below the larynx, the airways can be subdivided into three components: 1) the conducting airways consisting of the trachea, bronchi, and ending with the terminal bronchioles; 2) the transitional airways, consisting of respiratory bronchioles where gas is conducted and some gas exchange occurs; 3) the alveolar ducts, sacs, and alveoli, where gas exchange takes place with the pulmonary capillary blood.

The trachea, about 2.0–2.5 cm in diameter and nearly 11 cm long in the adult, extends from the level of the 6th cervical vertebra to the 5th thoracic vertebra. The trachea divides at the level of the carina, forming the right and left mainstem bronchi. The right and left mainstem bronchi further subdivide into lobar bronchi, then into subsegmental bronchi. The larger airways divide into even smaller airways similar to the branching of the roots of a tree. Collectively, the trachea and branching airways are commonly referred to as the tracheobronchial tree.

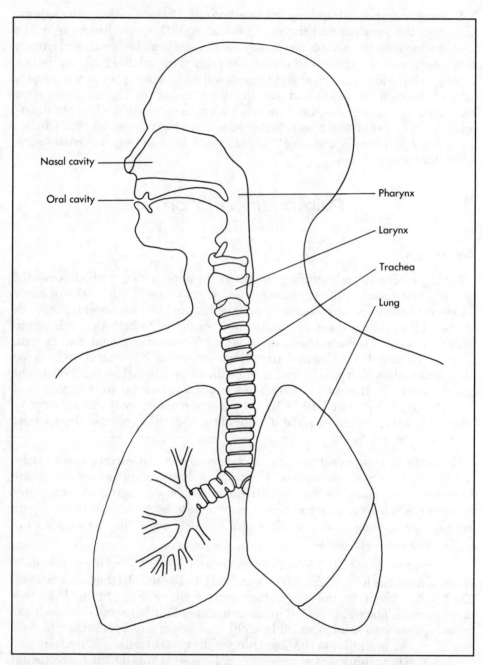

Figure 1-1   The respiratory tract. (From Dail, D.H.: Anatomy of the respiratory system, in Moser, K.M., Spragg, R.G. (eds), Respiratory Emergencies, 2nd ed., C.V. Mosby Co., St. Louis, 1982.)

Each division or generation of airways continues dividing until the air reaches the alveoli, the smallest division in the lungs. From the trachea to the alveoli the airway divides into approximately 23 generations or groups of branching airways in the adult (Fig. 1-2).

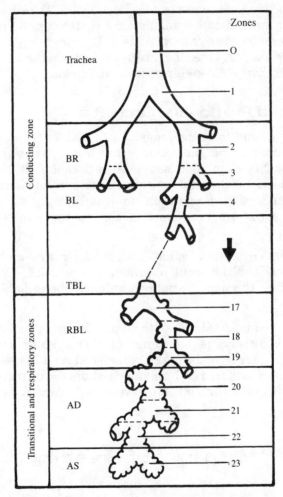

Figure 1-2   Subdivisions of the respiratory tract. BR, bronchus; BL, bronchiole; TBL, terminal bronchiole; RBL, respiratory bronchiole; AD, alveolar duct; AS, alveolar space.

Smooth muscle is located in the airway walls throughout most of the tracheobronchial tree although it varies in its location with the size of the airway. In the trachea and large bronchi, a band of muscle connects the opening of U-shaped cartilages that support the airway. As the airway size decreases, the smooth muscle becomes progressively more prominent with muscle fibers spiraling in both directions crisscrossing in the walls. Therefore, the effect of smooth muscle contraction (bronchospasm) is more significant distal to the trachea and large bronchi and will decrease airway diameter and length in these more peripheral airways. Smooth muscle has been identified in airway walls to the level of the respiratory bronchioles.

Ciliated columnar epithelial cells line nearly all of the respiratory tract below the larynx to the level of the respiratory bronchioles. The cilia that border the columnar epithelium constantly undulate in a rhythmic pattern similar to what is seen as the wind blows over a wheat field. This process removes most of the particles and debris that enter the airways. The escalator-like action of these cells does an effective job of keeping the airway clean.

Bronchial and Pulmonary Circulation

Blood supply to and from the lungs can be divided into two components: bronchial circulation and pulmonary circulation. Arterial blood flowing through the bronchial circulation is supplied by the aorta. Bronchial circulation is but one component of the total systemic circulation, and it serves to meet the metabolic demands of the lung tissue. Bronchial circulation supplies blood to and from the entire tracheo-bronchial tree to the level of the terminal bronchioles.

The pulmonary circulation begins in the right ventricle and ends in the left atrium, and supplies blood to the respiratory bronchioles, alveolar ducts and alveoli. Blood flow through the pulmonary circulation allows gas exchange to occur.

Some of the blood in capillaries of the bronchial and pulmonary circulation mix at the level of airways near the terminal and respiratory bronchioles. Most of the venous drainage from the intermixing blood empties into the left atrium, contributing in part to the normal anatomical shunt (blood traveling from right side of heart to left side without being oxygenated by the lung).

Mechanics of Breathing

The Chest Wall

The human thorax is rigid and structured to protect the vital organs contained within, yet flexible and pliable enough to permit chest expansion with breathing. The bones, cartilage and supportive tissue provide rigidity and strength to the thorax while the numerous points of articulation allow significant changes in size and shape. The 12 pairs of ribs provide the structural foundation of the chest (Fig. 1-3).

During inspiration, the chest and lungs expand in all three planes: antero-posterior, transverse, and longitudinal. The three-dimensional increase in the size of the chest occurs because the ribs move anteriorly, upward, and spread apart as a result of the contraction of the diaphragm and accessory muscles of inspiration.

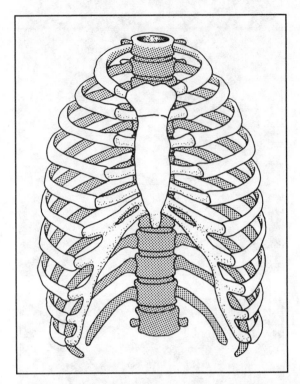

Figure 1-3   Rib formation of the chest cage. (From Dail, D.H.: Anatomy of the respiratory system, in Moser, K.M., Spragg, R.G. (eds), Respiratory Emergencies, 2nd ed., C.V. Mosby Co., St. Louis, 1982.)

Muscles of Respiration

The muscles used in breathing can be divided into two components, primary and accessory (see Fig. 1-5). The primary muscle of respiration is the diaphragm which is composed of two dome-shaped hemidiaphragms that form the floor of the thorax and separate the thorax from the abdomen. During inspiration, the diaphragm contracts and flattens and descends toward the abdomen. Diaphragmatic contraction causes the longitudinal lung size to increase. During exhalation, the diaphragm relaxes and ascends while returning to its resting, dome-shaped configuration (Fig. 1-4).

Accessory muscles of breathing, located in the neck and upper part of the chest, can assist the diaphragm in increasing thoracic volume. Accessory muscles of breathing include sternocleidomastoid, trapezius, intercostal, and rhomboid muscles. These muscles normally are not active during relaxed breathing but begin participating in breathing with activity or when the resistance to air movement into the thorax is increased. Rapid breathing with

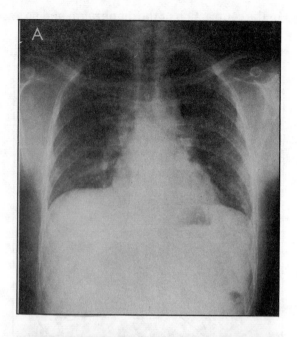

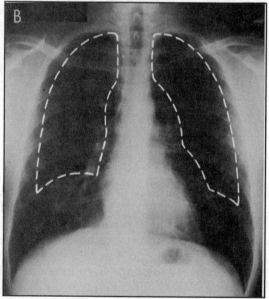

Figure 1-4 Roentgenogram of same chest in full expiration (A) and full inspiration (B). Dashed white line in B is outline of lungs in full expiration (as in A). (From Comroe, J.H.: Physiology of Respiration, 2nd ed., Year Book Medical Publishers, Chicago, 1974.)

exercise, cardiopulmonary diseases or any problem that increases the work of breathing, often causes the accessory muscles of breathing to become active to augment ventilation. The accessory muscles can increase the magnitude of chest expansion and lung size that occurs during inspiration (Fig. 1-5).

The abdominal muscles usually do not participate actively in relaxed breathing; however, during forced exhalation, rapid breathing, exercise, coughing, or sneezing, the abdominal muscles play an important part in providing maximum function. They are important especially in the post-operative patient who must use them to generate an effective cough.

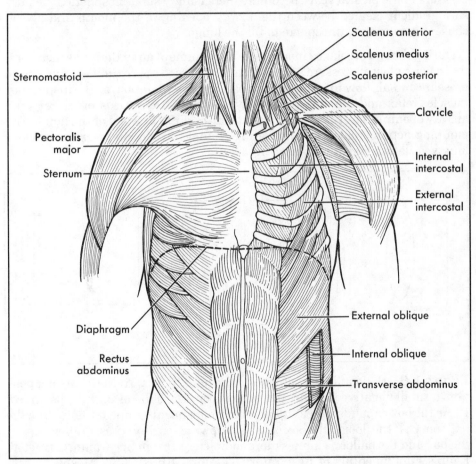

Figure 1-5   The muscles of ventilation. (From Spearman, C.B., et al: Egan's Fundamentals of Respiratory Therapy, 4th ed., C.V. Mosby Co., St. Louis, 1982.)

Forces and Flow Patterns

From a mechanical point of view, the lungs and surrounding chest wall form the ventilatory apparatus that is similar in function to a pump. The chest wall and lungs are separated by the parietal and visceral pleura. The pressure in the pleural space is referred to as the pleural pressure and varies during breathing. During the end of relaxed expiration, the lung recoils inwardly like a rubber band, returning to its original position after stretching. The recoil of the chest wall is directed outwardly. These opposing forces generate a subatmospheric pressure of approximately 5 cm of water that varies in magnitude throughout each breathing cycle. In the resting state, when there is no air flow in or out of the lungs, the airway resistance is zero and the pressure along the entire airway from the mouth to the alveoli is nearly equal to atmospheric pressure. During inspiration, the diaphragm contracts and the lung expands as a result of the pressure in the pleural space becoming increasingly subatmospheric. The pressure gradient created between the airway opening of the mouth and alveoli causes air from the atmosphere to fill the lungs.

During the end of relaxed inspiration, the volume of air in the lungs increases; this causes pleural pressure and alveolar pressure to approximate atmospheric pressure and air flow into the lung stops. During exhalation, as the inspiratory muscles relax and the lung recoils, alveolar pressure exceeds pressure at the airway opening. The pressure gradient causes air to flow out of the lungs. The pumping action created by alternating changes in pleural pressure provides lung ventilation essential to life (Fig. 1-6).

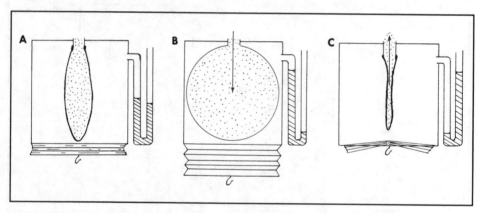

Figure 1-6   Balloon in a box model of the lung-thorax. **A,** In the resting position, a small negative pressure in the box keeps the balloon slightly distended. **B,** As the box expands the cavity becomes more negative and air flows into the balloon. **C,** If the floor of the box is pushed upward, positive pressure develops in the box and the balloon empties more completely. (From Spearman, C.B., et al: Egan's Fundamentals of Respiratory Therapy, 4th ed., C.V. Mosby Co., St. Louis)

Sounds in Normal Airways

After the age of 2 years, the lungs contain more than 300 million alveoli. If the alveoli were placed next to each other on a flat surface, they would cover an area between 50 and 100 m^2, about the size of a tennis court. In contrast, the trachea has a cross-sectional area of only 3–5 cm^2. Air passing through the trachea is rapid and turbulent, thereby creating more audible sounds as the molecules of air bounce against the airway wall and against each other (see Fig. 1–7). As the volume of air inhaled passes through the ever-branching airways to the alveoli, the airflow becomes more laminar since the sum total of the diameters of each generation increases exponentially. Peripherally in the lung, the volume of inhaled gas is "spread out" over many airways and airflow is slower and less turbulent.

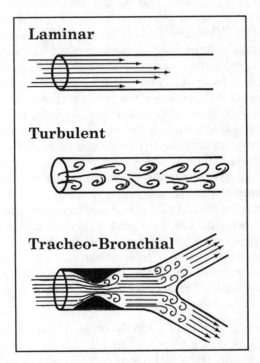

Figure 1-7   Types of air flow. In smooth, straight tubes, turbulent flow occurs only at high velocities; these usually occur only in large tubes, such as the main bronchi and trachea, especially when there is hyperpnea. The flow rate in the fine tubes is very low because the total air flow is divided among hundreds of thousands of tubes. However, eddy formation may occur at each branching of the tracheobronchial tree, and the pressure required for eddy flow is approximately the same as for turbulent flow. Turbulence (at low flow rates) or eddy formation is particularly apt to occur where there are irregularities in the tubes, such as those caused by mucus, exudate, tumor or foreign bodies or partial closure of the glottis. Sometimes air flow is a combination of laminar and turbulent flow with eddy formation. (Reproduced with permission from Forester, R.E. II, et. al.: The Lung: Physiologic Basis of Pulmonary Function Test, 3rd ed., Year Book Medical Publishers, Chicago, 1986.)

Physiology of Respiration

Lung Volumes and Capacities

The volume of air occupying the lungs can be subdivided into lung volumes and capacities that can be measured directly by spirometry and indirectly by gas dilution techniques (Fig. 1–8). During normal breathing, the volume of air entering the lungs during inspiration and leaving the lungs during exhalation is the tidal volume (VT). The sum of all the inhaled air measured over a minute is the inspiratory minute volume ($\dot{V}_I$) and the sum of all the exhaled air measured over a minute is the expiratory minute volume ($\dot{V}_E$). The maximum volume of air that can be inhaled from the end of a resting inhaled volume is the inspiratory reserve volume (IRV). The sum of the tidal volume and inspiratory reserve volume compartments comprise the inspiratory capacity (IC). This is achieved from a maximal inhaled volume originating from the end of a resting exhaled tidal volume. The maximum volume of air exhaled from the end of a normal resting exhaled tidal volume is the expiratory reserve volume (ERV). The volume of air remaining in the lungs after maximal exhalation is the residual volume (RV). The sum of the expiratory reserve volume and the residual volume compartments comprise the functional residual capacity (FRC). The volume of air in the lungs following maximal inspiration is the total lung capacity (TLC). The maximal volume of air exhaled from the lungs after a maximal inspiration is the vital capacity (VC) for exhalation and the maximum volume of air inhaled following maximal exhalation is the vital capacity (VC) for inspiration. Normally the VC for inspiration and exhalation are equivalent. The sum of the IRV, TV and ERV components comprise the VC.

The resting level and volume of air in the lungs is determined by the balance between the elastic, recoiling forces of the lungs, which tend to decrease the volume of the lungs; and, the elastic, recoiling forces of the chest wall, which tend to increase the volume. The resting volume in the lungs can be altered by many factors. As the lungs lose elasticity with aging, or with emphysema, the FRC increases. When lung expandability decreases, as in pulmonary fibrosis, the FRC decreases. The FRC also diminishes when there is a change from the erect position to the supine position, which is caused by a shift of the gravitational position, resulting in an impingement of the abdomen on the diaphragm.

Gas Exchange

The major function of the lungs is to provide oxygen to, and remove carbon dioxide from, the blood flowing through the pulmonary capillaries. During breathing, alveolar air and pulmonary capillary blood come into intimate contact separated only by an ultrathin alveolar-capillary membrane.

Blood leaving the right ventricle flows through the pulmonary capillaries richly perfusing the alveoli. Some of the oxygen leaves the alveoli and diffuses across the alveolar-capillary membrane into the blood while some of the carbon

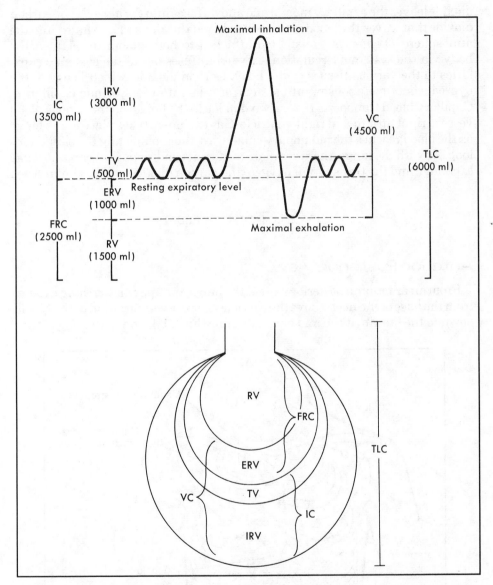

Figure 1-8 Lung capacities and volumes. Representation of a normal spirogram and the divisions of lung volumes and capacities. Numbers shown are for comparison for an average sized, young adult. (From Spearman, C.B., et al: Egan's Fundamentals of Respiratory Therapy, 4th ed., C.V. Mosby Co., St. Louis, 1982.)

dioxide leaves the capillary membrane and diffuses into the alveoli. The carbon dioxide that leaves the blood via the alveoli and the airways is exhaled into the atmosphere. Oxygen is transported attached to hemoglobin throughout the body via the systemic circulation. Oxygen diffuses out of the systemic capillaries to the various tissues of the body. Carbon dioxide, which is one of the byproducts of metabolism, diffuses out of cells into the systemic capillaries. Capillary blood transports the carbon dioxide to the lungs via the venous blood vessels, right atrium and right ventricle. Gas exchange takes place in the lungs as the blood reaches the pulmonary capillaries, thus completing the circulatory loop. As with the lungs, there are many different conditions that can affect gas exchange and the transport of oxygen and carbon dioxide at the cellular level.

Chest Topography

Anterior-Posterior View

From an anterior to posterior view of the lungs, the apex of each lung extends from the base of the neck above the clavicle near the vertebral end of the 1st rib, down to the 6th rib at the mid-clavicular line (Figs. 1-9 and 1-10).

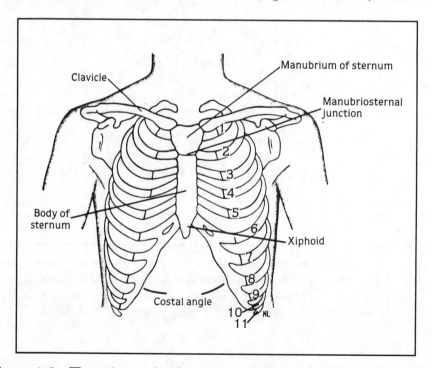

Figure 1-9   Thoracic cage landmarks on anterior chest. (From Wilkins, R.L., Sheldon, R.L., and Krider, S.J.: Clinical Assessment in Respiratory Care, C.V. Mosby Co., St. Louis, 1985.)

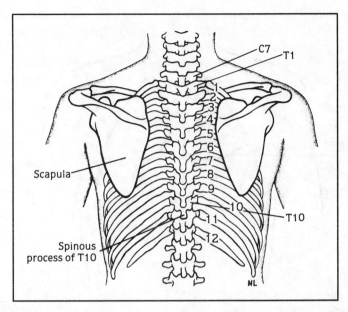

Figure 1-10   Thoracic cage landmarks on posterior chest. (From Wilkins, R.L., Sheldon, R.L., and Krider, S.J.: Clinical Assessment in Respiratory Care, C.V. Mosby Co., St. Louis, 1985.)

The right lung is divided into the upper and middle lobe by the horizontal fissure which begins near the 4th rib anteriorly at the midsternal line and continues laterally to the 5th rib at the midaxillary line. The oblique fissure of the right lung separates the lower lobe from the upper and middle lobe. It extends from the 6th rib anteriorly at the midclavicular line ascending to the 4th rib posteriorly (Figs. 1-11 and 1-12). The oblique fissure for the left lung separates the lower lobe from the upper lobe. It occupies a similar position as the right oblique fissure. The breath sounds of the upper lobes of both lungs and the right middle lobe dominate the auscultation findings heard on the anterior chest.

Posterior-Anterior View

From a posterior to anterior view the lungs are divided into upper and lower lobes by the oblique fissure. It originates near the 4th rib or at T-3 at the midspinal line and extends anteriorly to the level of the 6th rib. The lower lobes dominate the surface area of the posterior chest wall. The upper lobes can be auscultated posteriorly above the midlevel of the scapula.

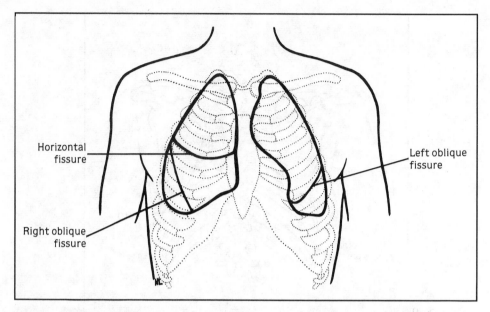

Figure 1-11   Topographic position of lung fissures on anterior chest. (From Wilkins, R.L., Sheldon, R.L., and Krider, S.J.: Clinical Assessment in Respiratory Care, C.V. Mosby Co., St. Louis, 1985.)

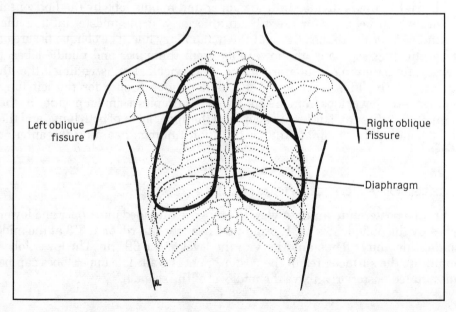

Figure 1-12   Topographic position of lung fissures on posterior chest. (From Wilkins, R.L., Sheldon, R.L., and Krider, S.J.: Clinical Assessment in Respiratory Care, C.V. Mosby Co., St. Louis, 1985.)

Alterations in the Lungs with Chest Disease

Chest diseases can be classified into either restrictive or obstructive lung disorders, or a combination of the two. Restrictive lung diseases cause a reduction in lung volume and an increase in lung tissue density. Obstructive lung disorders primarily affect the airways and alveoli, resulting in diminished airflow. Air trapping often occurs resulting in hyperinflation of the distal air spaces and a decrease in lung tissue density.

Restrictive and obstructive lung diseases cause dramatic changes in pulmonary anatomy and physiology. Many of these changes can be detected on physical examination including significant alterations in lung sounds, as will be discussed in subsequent chapters.

Neonatal Anatomy and Physiology*

The infant has several developmental differences in the structure and function of the lung. The lung develops and grows continuously from fetal life through childhood. The understanding of this growth and development of the lung is helpful to interpret the pulmonary signs identified by physical examination.

Pulmonary Anatomy

The trachea of the newborn is funnel shaped, wider at the larynx and more narrow toward the carina. It becomes cylindrical as the infant grows. The trachea's greatest rate of growth occurs between 1 month and 4 years of age. The major growth of the airways is during the 10th to 14th week of gestation when 70% of the bronchial tree is established. However, there are 2–4 generations of airways and large numbers of branches of these airways that will develop between the 24th week of gestation and term.

The surface area of the lung rapidly increases during the last trimester of pregnancy and during infancy. The surface area of the lung increases from approximately 1 m² at 28 weeks gestational age to about 4 m² at term. The term infant's lung has approximately 55 million alveoli. This number will increase rapidly until the child's lung has approximately 300 million alveoli at about 2 years of age. The shape of the alveoli changes from the sacular-like structures to the mature decahedronic structure of the adult over the first 4–6 years of life.

Pulmonary Circulation

The newborn infant has the potential for several intracardiac and extracardiac shunts. First, the ductus arteriosus is patent for the first 2–3 days of life. The ductus arteriosus is a large vessel that is patent during fetal circulation to allow blood to flow from the pulmonary artery to the aorta, bypassing the lung. After

*Written by Douglas D. Deming.

birth, normally it will close in response to the increased blood PO_2. The foramen ovale is an opening in the interatrial septum that opens to allow blood to flow into the left atrium from the right atrium. It is functionally (but not anatomically) closed by the left atrial pressure being greater than the right atrial pressure. Finally, the infant frequently has intrapulmonary shunts.

During intrauterine life, the infant shunts blood away from the lungs through the patent ductus arteriosus and the foramen ovale. The shunting occurs because the pulmonary vascular resistance (PVR) is higher than the systemic vascular resistance (SVR). During the period of transitional circulation after delivery, the PVR decreases because the infant has taken his first breath and gas has expanded the lung. Concomitantly, the SVR increases because the placenta has been removed from the systemic circulation. During this transitional period the resistance of the two vascular beds is approximately equal with the SVR being slightly higher than the PVR. Any stimulus that causes a rise in the PVR has the potential to again cause a right to left shunt through either the foramen ovale or the ductus arteriosus (e.g., Persistent Pulmonary Hypertension).

After the infant enters the period of neonatal circulation, the SVR will be greater than the PVR. The PVR will decrease rapidly during the first 4–6 weeks of life and then slowly decrease until approximately 3 years of age when it achieves adult values. The SVR increases progressively throughout life with the greatest increase having occurred before 10 years of age.

Mechanical Properties of the Chest Wall and Lung

One of the most profound differences between the adult and infant is in the mechanics of the respiratory system which is comprised of the chest wall and the lung.

The very compliant chest wall of the newborn allows for the necessary compression needed to permit the infant to pass from the uterus through the vaginal canal at birth. However, this means that the compliance of the chest wall is close to the compliance of the lung. This fact raises two issues that must be considered when evaluating the infant. First, the outward force of the chest wall is less resulting in a lower functional residual capacity. Second, any of a variety of diseases can cause a fall in the compliance of the lung that will create the mechanical disadvantage of the chest wall being more compliant than the lung (e.g., retractions in Respiratory Distress Syndrome).

Additionally, the lung of the infant is less compliant than the adult. This is probably because the infant's functional residual capacity is maintained at a lower percent of total lung capacity. However, the result of this higher chest wall compliance, lower lung compliance, and lower functional residual capacity is manifested by the infant as rapid shallow breathing.

As in the adult, the infant's diaphragm is the major source of power for gas movement into the lung. The differences are in the support by the chest wall and the use of accessory muscles of respiration. In the adult, during inspiration, the thoracic cavity increases longitudinally from top to bottom as well as circumferentially. Whereas, the infant's thoracic cavity increases much more longitudinally in the top to bottom direction than it does circumferentially. Because there is less support of the chest wall by the accessory muscles, the greater expansion of the infant's lung occurs at the bases.

The infant's tidal breathing occurs at a lower FRC than the adult's therefore, the infant's closing volume (that volume of the lung where airways close) is in the mid-tidal volume range. The infant compensates for this by taking shallow rapid breaths.

Gas Transport

The presence of hemoglobin F changes the infant's ability to transport oxygen from the lung to the tissues. The oxygen dissociation curve for hemoglobin F is to the left of the curve for hemoglobin A. This means that the infant's red blood cells with hemoglobin F will attach to oxygen more readily and will release oxygen less readily to the tissues than would cells with hemoglobin A.

Chest Topography

There is little change in the topography of the lung from fetus to infant to adult. However, the external chest wall does change its shape from being round to ovoid in the transverse plane (see Fig. 1–13).

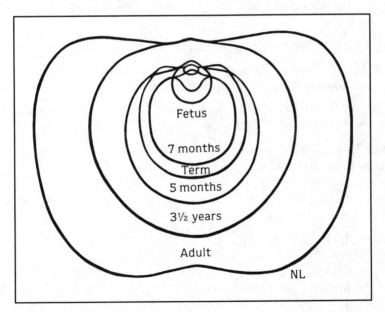

Figure 1-13   Changes in anteroposterior chest configuration with age. (From Wilkins, R.L., Sheldon, R.L., and Krider, S.J.: Clinical Assessment in Respiratory Care, C.V. Mosby Co., St. Louis, 1985.)

The cross-sectional area of the thoracic cavity in the adult is fairly equal from base to apex. Whereas, the infant's cross-sectional area is much larger at the base than at the apex. These differences tend to make the infant's chest appear more "bell shaped" than an adult's.

When the infant's chest is viewed from the side it appears to have a proportionally greater A-P diameter than an adult's. Also, during the respiratory cycle the majority of the infant's chest wall movement is an anterior-posterior motion of the anterior chest wall rather than a uniform circumferential expansion around the chest observed in adults.

Bibliography

Burton, G.G. and Hodgkin, J.E.: *Respiratory Care, A Guide to Clinical Practice,* ed. 2, Philadelphia, 1984, J.B. Lippincott Co.

Cherniack, R.M. and Cherniack, L.: *Respiration in Health and Disease,* ed. 3, Philadelphia, 1983, W.B. Saunders Co.

Green, J.F.: *Fundamental Cardiovascular and Pulmonary Physiology,* ed. 2, Philadelphia, 1987, Lea & Febiger.

Johnson, T.R., Moore, W.M., and Jeffries, J.E.: *Children Are Different: Developmental Physiology,* ed. 2, Columbus, 1978, Ross Laboratories.

Martin, L.: *Pulmonary Physiology in Clinical Practice,* St. Louis, 1987, C.V. Mosby Co.

Murray, J.F.: *The Normal Lung,* ed. 2, Philadelphia, 1986, W. B. Saunders Co.

Netter, F.H.: *Respiratory System: The Ciba Collection of Medical Illustration, Vol. 7,* New Jersey, 1979, Ciba Pharmaceutical Co.

Spearman, C.B., Sheldon, R.L., and Egan, D.F.: *Egan's Fundamentals of Respiratory Therapy,* ed. 4, St. Louis, 1982, C.V. Mosby Co.

Thibeault, D.W., and Gregory, G.A.: *Neonatal Pulmonary Care,* ed. 2, Norwalk, 1986, Appleton-Century-Crofts.

CHAPTER
2
Clinical Assessment of the Pulmonary Patient

David B. Martin

Objectives

After reading this chapter, the learner should be able to recognize and describe:

1. The common symptoms of pulmonary disease and their significant characteristics to identify in the interview.

2. Correct techniques for inspection, palpation, percussion and auscultation of the chest.

3. Common causes for abnormalities identified during physical examination of the patient with pulmonary disease.

4. The value of other assessment adjuncts including chest roentgenograms, pulmonary function testing, and arterial blood gases.

Anyone who auscultates patients should understand how pulmonary assessment fits into the overall picture. With this in mind, this chapter provides an overview of the basic knowledge needed to properly assess the patient with pulmonary disease. The initial assessment, usually performed by a physician, requires a careful history, a detailed physical examination, a chest film, and a judgment pertaining to the acuteness and activity of the disease. Once the initial assessment is made, subsequent assessments will need to be performed by other health care practitioners to evaluate the patient's response to therapy. Valuable adjuncts to the assessment include arterial blood gas analysis, sputum evaluation, pulmonary function testing, and possibly bronchoscopy. Each assessment often requires usage of a variety of the components described in this chapter.

The Medical History

The initial medical history is an account of the events in the patient's life that have relevance to his physical and mental health. The information obtained by interviewing a patient with a respiratory complaint is complete only with careful probing. The fundamental principles of interviewing the pulmonary patient are no different than other medical histories. These principles include careful listening and questioning, in association with skillful observation. The initial and subsequent interviews usually center around a discussion of the patient's chief complaints or symptoms. There are several *symptoms* that are common in patients with cardiopulmonary disease.

Cough

Cough is required for self cleansing of the airways but may be secondary to inflammation or irritation of the airway lining. This symptom readily brings attention to the lungs. An acute cough is difficult for the patient to ignore, in contrast to a chronic cough which the patient may feel is customary or habit. This is particularly true of the smoker's cough. The typical smoker often has a daily ritual of morning cigarette, newspaper, coffee, and 3 or 4 minutes of productive coughing.

Other factors to be considered besides the acuteness or chronicity of the cough are the circumstances of the cough: does the cough only occur with exercise, weather changes, or exposure to suspected allergenic materials? This type of coughing might occur in a patient with reversible bronchospasm or asthma. Coughing with a change in body position may suggest a chronic bronchitis or bronchogenic carcinoma.

The character of the cough, whether it be dry or productive, is also of importance. A dry cough, often described by clinicians as barking (seal-like), brassy, or hoarse usually is indicative of an acute irritative process. With this description, inhalation of noxious fumes, or possibly an allergy leading to an irritated hypopharynx and post nasal drip may be the cause. Most likely, however, a simple, viral infection is the cause. See Table 2-1 for a description of the terms used to describe coughing and their possible significance.

Table 2-1.   Terms Used to Describe Coughing*

Description	Possible Causes
Barking	Epiglottal disease, croup, influenza, laryngotracheal bronchitis
Brassy or hoarse	Laryngitis, laryngeal paralysis, laryngotracheal bronchitis, pressure on recurrent laryngeal nerve, mediastinal tumor, aortic aneurysm, left atrial enlargement
Inspiratory stridor	Tracheal or mainstem bronchial obstruction, croup, epiglottitis
Wheezy	Bronchospasm, asthma, cystic fibrosis
Dry	Viral infections, inhalation of irritant gases, interstitial lung diseases, tumor, pleural effusion, cardiac condition, nervous habit, radiation therapy, chemotherapy
Dry progressing to productive	Atypical and mycoplasmal pneumonia. Legionnaires' disease, pulmonary embolus and edema, lung abscess, asthma, silicosis, emphysema (late in disease)
Chronic productive	Bronchiectasis, chronic bronchitis, lung abscess, asthma, fungal infections, bacterial pneumonias, tuberculosis
Inadequate	Debility, weakness, oversedation, pain, poor motivation
Paroxysmal (especially at night)	Aspiration, asthma, left heart failure
Morning	Chronic bronchitis, smoking
Afternoon and evening	Exposure to irritants during the day
Associated with lying down or position change	Bronchiectasis, left heart failure, chronic postnasal drip or sinusitis, gastroesophageal reflux with aspiration
Associated with eating or drinking	Neuromuscular disease of the upper airway, esophageal problems

*From Wilkins, R.L., Sheldon, R.L., and Krider, S.J.: Clinical assessment in respiratory care, St. Louis, 1985, The C. V. Mosby Co.

A neoplasm (abnormal formation of tissue) in the respiratory tree, benign or malignant, would lead to coughing by direct mechanical irritation of the respiratory tissues and thus cough receptor stimulation.

A productive cough is a cough that produces pulmonary secretions; this is recognized easily by its longer duration and distinctive sound. A productive cough persisting for months or years which is worse in the morning is suggestive of chronic bronchitis. This would especially be true if it is associated with a smoking history. Bronchiectasis, an insidious disease causing permanent dilatation of the bronchial tubes, also is associated with chronic cough and sputum production. Frequently, a profuse amount of secretions, e.g., 2–3 cupfuls of phlegm, is produced each day.

Sputum with an acute productive cough may be purulent (pus containing), or non purulent, i.e., the silicone-like plugs produced by the typical asthmatic (see Table 2–2). Acute purulence suggests infection. A sample of the sputum should be gram stained and analyzed under the microscope for the presence of pus cells and bacteria. Greater than 25 leukocytes per high power field (hpf) is suggestive of infection. Under hpf, a ratio of greater than 10/1 epithelial cells to pus cells is highly suggestive of oral contamination. The gram stain obtained in this situation might be unreliable since the analyzed sample may represent oral rather than lung secretions. The technician or pathologist reading the slide always should provide this ratio.

Table 2-2.   Presumptive Sputum Analysis*

Appearance of Sputum	Possible Causes
Mucoid	Bronchial asthma (small silicone-like bronchial casts), Legionnaires' disease (grayish), pulmonary tuberculosis, emphysema, neoplasms, and early chronic bronchitis
Mucopurulent	Above and infection, pneumonias, cystic fibrosis
Purulent	
Yellow or green copious	Bronchiectasis (separates into layers) advanced chronic bronchitis, pseudomonas pneumonia
Apple, green, thick	Haemophilus influenzae pneumonia
Pink, thin, blood streaked	Streptococcal pneumonia, staphylococcal pneumonia
Red currant jelly	Klebsiella pneumonia
Rusty	Pneumococcal pneumonia
Foul odor	Lung abscess, bronchiectasis, anaerobic infections, aspiration
Sand or small stone	Broncholithiasis, aspiration of foreign material
Black	Smoke or coal dust inhalation
Frothy white or pink	Pulmonary edema
Blood streaked or frankly bloody (hemoptysis)	*Pulmonary:* Embolism with infarction, pneumonias, bronchiectasis, neoplasm, tuberculosis, abscess, trauma, arteriovenous malformation, aspiration of a foreign body, pulmonary hypertension
	Cardiac: Mitral valve disease, pulmonary edema
	Systemic: Coagulation disorders, Wegener's granulomatosis, Goodpasture's syndrome, sarcoidosis
	Other: Emesis, oropharyngeal bleed rather than true hemoptysis

*From Wilkins, R.L., Sheldon, R.L., and Krider, S.J.: Clinical assessment in respiratory care, St. Louis, 1985, The C. V. Mosby Co.

Other important information obtained by the reliable gram stain include the size and shape of the bacteria seen and the presence of fungi. A wet-mount preparation or Wright stain to differentiate between the presence of eosinophils and neutrophils can be helpful in determining whether the cough is due to an allergic disorder or infection. Numerous eosinophils in a sputum specimen can be indicative of an allergic response, parasitic infestation, or other serious pulmonary disorder.

Dyspnea

Dyspnea, or literally "difficult breathing" as perceived by the patient, is a symptom that is likely to be reported by the patient as "smothering," "quickly out of breath," a "tightness in the chest," or "can't take a deep breath." Occasionally the patient may appear to be short of breath but will not complain of difficult breathing when asked. Dyspnea can be classified as "dyspnea at rest," "with exertion only," with "laying down" (orthopnea) or as "awakening at night" with dyspnea (paroxysmal nocturnal dyspnea).

The etiology of dyspnea is potentially far reaching and ranges from physiologic, that associated with physical exertion, to the dyspnea of cardiac failure as output from the left ventricle fails to keep up with metabolic needs. Dyspnea may also be psychogenic, as when associated with hysterical hyperventilation.

In patients with lung disease, dyspnea usually is due to a disorder which results in an increased work of breathing, such as restrictive defects that decrease the compliance of the lungs or chest wall, or obstructive defects with partial airways obstruction (see Table 2–3). Restrictive lung disease can lead to intense dyspnea, especially with exertion. Obstructive defects lead to dyspnea due to the increased resistance to air movement through the airways. This increases the work of breathing and causes the patient to feel dyspneic.

Table 2-3.   Some Diseases and Symptoms Associated with Dyspnea*

Diseases	Dyspnea	Associated Symptoms
Emphysema	Predominant symptom, insidious onset, exertional, recumbent, may be relieved by coughing	Coughing in advanced stages
Asthma	Episodic, may be exertional, symptom-free between attacks	Wheezing, productive coughing, tightness in chest
Chronic bronchitis	In advanced stages or with infection	Chronic, productive coughing
Upper airway obstruction	Severity is dependent on size of object/tumor, amount of edema	Coughing, possible dull or pleuritic pain
Pulmonary congestion		
Acute	Abrupt, slow regression	Tachypnea, "cardiac wheeze," coughing
Chronic	Gradual onset over time with orthopnea, paroxysmal nocturnal dyspnea	Tachypnea, "cardiac wheeze," coughing
Pneumothorax	Moderate to severe	Sudden and sharp pleuritic pain
Pleural effusion	Usually present	Possible pleuritis dull pain
Chest wall deformities	Only in severe deformities	
Obesity, Pickwickian syndrome	Only on exertion	
Bacterial pneumonia	Exertional	Productive cough, pleuritic pain
Lung abscess	Frequent	Productive cough, pleuritic pain
Tuberculosis	Advanced cases	Productive cough, pleuritic pain
Diffuse lung disease (Hamman-Rich syndrome)	Present	Variable depending on disease; rate of respiration is increased
Pulmonary fibrosis		
Nonchemical (includes dusts allergens)	Progressive, exertional	Tachypnea, dry cough progressing to productive wheezing, pain
Chemical	Present	Wheezing, coughing, pain

*From Wilkins, R.L., Sheldon, R.L., and Krider, S.J.: Clinical assessment in respiratory care, St. Louis, 1985, The C. V. Mosby Co.

Hemoptysis

Hemoptysis, coughing up blood, is particularly alarming to the individual who experiences it. Usually the complaint is "blood tinged sputum." This symptom should never be ignored since serious lung or cardiac disorders, (i.e., bronchogenic cancer, tuberculosis, pulmonary embolism, mitral stenosis), can cause hemoptysis. It is also important to determine whether the lungs actually are the source of the blood reported (see Table 2-4). A trivial nosebleed or serious esophageal variceal bleeding may be erroneously reported as hemoptysis.

Table 2-4.   Distinguishing Characteristics of Hemoptysis and Hematemesis*

Characteristics	Hemoptysis	Hematemesis
History	Cardiopulmonary disease	Gastrointestinal disease
Patient statement	Coughed from lungs	Vomited from stomach
Blood		
pH	Alkaline	Acid
Color	Bright red	Dark (coffee grounds)
		Clotted
Froth	May be present	Absent
Mixed with	Sputum	Food
Associated symptoms	Dyspnea, pain or tickling sensation in chest	Nausea, pain referred to stomach

*From Wilkins, R.L., Sheldon, R.L., and Krider, S.J.: Clinical assessment in respiratory care, St. Louis, 1985, The C. V. Mosby Co.

Chest Pain

Chest pain is most often thought of as the cardinal symptom of cardiac disease but may be due to pulmonary disease as well. Usually chest pain associated with pulmonary disease is due to stimulation of pain fibers in the chest wall and/or parietal pleura. Pleuritic chest pain is associated with an inflamed parietal pleura and is predominantly present during inspiration and located laterally (see Table 2-5). The parietal pleura is innervated by intercostal nerves, and the pain is usually sharp, severe, and located at the site of the irritative process. Patients usually notice that the pain is lessened by lying on the affected side; which decreases movement of that side of the chest (autosplinting). This sign usually means involvement of the parietal pleura by such diseases as tuberculosis, pulmonary infarction, pneumonia, or spontaneous pneumothorax.

Table 2-5.   Causes and Characteristics of Chest Pain.*

Condition	Location and Characteristics	Etiology/precipitating factors	Associated findings
CHEST WALL PAIN			
Myalgia	Intercostal and pectoralis muscles Localized, dull aching Increases with movement Usually long lasting	Trauma, seizure, non-isometric and isometric exercise Persistent severe cough	Usually no visible erythema or ecchymosis with occult trauma
Chondro-ostealgia	Ribs and cartilages, precisely located (chondral pain in sternal area) Increases with pressure to area, movement, respiration, coughing Can be severe and disabling	Trauma (e.g., steering wheel, cardiopulmonary resuscitation) severe coughing in osteoporosis, tumor, myelocytic leukemia, systemic autoimmune disease, Tietze's syndrome	Rib fractures, chondral dislocations, periostitis, fever with some systemic causes
Neuralgia	Dermatome distribution Superficial tingling to deep burning pain	Thoracic spine disease, metastatic tumor, autoimmune and connective tissue disease	Specific changes on x-ray films, fever with infections
PLEURITIC AND PULMONARY PAIN			
Pleuritis (pleurisy)	Pleura, usually well localized Sharp, stabbing, raw, burning Often rapid onset, increased by inspiration, coughing, laughing, hiccuping	Infection/inflammation of pleura, trauma, autoimmune and connective tissue disease	Fever, productive cough, tachypnea, splinting of affected side
Pulmonary embolus and pulmonary infarction	Usually at base of lung, may radiate to abdomen or costal margins Stabbing, sudden onset, increased by inspiration	Immobilization, obesity, pelvic surgery	Symptoms vary with size of embolus Anxiety to panic Dyspnea, tachypnea, tachycardia, coughing with blood tinged to hemoptic sputum
Pneumothorax	Lateral thorax, well localized Sharp, tearing Sudden onset Increased by inspiration	Interstitial lung disease, bullous emphysema, asthma, idiopathic May follow deep inspiration, Valsalva maneuver, exercise, or occur at rest	Dyspnea, tachypnea, decreased breath sounds on affected side Mediastinal shift and jugular venous distention if tension pneumothorax develops
Tumors	May be localized or diffuse Constant, sharp, boring, or dull	Invasion of primary or metastatic tumor through parenchyma to parietal pleura, mesothelioma	Symptoms vary with type and location Evidence from x-ray films History of asbestos exposure
Pulmonary hypertension (primary)	Substernal, dull, aching similar to angina Related to stress and exertion	Unknown Seen most commonly in young females	Dyspnea, tachypnea, anxiety, syncope, jugular venous distention

Table 2-5. *(continued)*

Condition	Location and Characteristics	Etiology/precipitating factors	Associated findings
CARDIAC PAIN			
Angina pectoris	Substernal, may radiate to arms, shoulders, neck, and jaw Tightness to dull, heavy pressure-like pain not related to respiration Sudden onset, short duration	Coronary artery block- or spasm Hot, humid weather, large meals, intense emotion, exertion	Anxiety, feeling of impending doom, dyspnea, sweating, nausea Relieved by nitroglycerin and rest
Myocardial infarction	Substernal, radiating like angina Sudden crashing, viselike pain lasting minutes to hours		As above, disphoresis, vomiting Not relieved by nitro-glycerin or rest
Pericardial pain	Substernal or parasternal radiating to neck, shoulder, and epi-gastrium, (rarely to arms) Sharp, stabbing, inter-mittent Intensified by respiration and lying on left side	Inflammation of peri-cardium, infection, metastatic tumor, trauma, irradiation, autoimmune diseases	Pericardial friction rub Tachycardia, distended neck veins, paradoxical pulse with tamponade, dyspnea
MEDIASTINAL PAIN			
Esophageal	Substernal, retrosternal, epigastric Radiates toward shoulders Deep buring pain Sudden, tearing pain	Esophagitis aggravated by bending over, lying down, smoking, inges-tion of coffee/fats/ large meals Esophageal spasm Esophageal tear	Regurgitation of sour-tasting acid secretions relieved by antacids or may be relieved by nitroglycerin Hematemesis, shock
Dissecting aortic aneurysm	Tearing midline chest or posterior thoracic pain Sudden onset, may last hours	Blunt trauma, hyperten-sion, inflammatory or degenerative diseases	May have lower blood pressure in legs or one arm, paralysis, murmur of aortic insufficiency, paradoxical pulse, hypertension, shock, death
Tracheobronchitis	Substernal burning dis-comfort May be referred to anterior chest	Acute viral infections, prolonged cigarette smoking	Cough may or may not be productive May have fever with infection
Other causes	Retrosternal or epigastric pain or burning Vague tightness to severe crushing	Referred abdominal pain: hiatal hernia, peptic ulcer, gallbladder Hyperventilation syndrome	Symptoms vary with disease Respiratory distress, tachypnea, diaphoresis, numbness of fingers and around mouth Respiratory alkalosis

*From Wilkins, R.L., Sheldon, R.L., and Krider, S.J.: Clinical assessment in respiratory care, St. Louis, 1985, The C. V. Mosby Co.

Airway inflamation may lead to a pain described as a burning sensation and usually is pinpointed as retrosternal. Such causes of tracheal irritation as viral tracheitis, exposure to extreme cold, and inhalation of noxious fumes lead to pain of this type.

Other important factors to be included in the pulmonary history are the presence or absence of hoarseness, wheezing, or peripheral edema of the lower extremities. Peripheral edema is common in patients with right-sided heart failure due to a chronic increase in pulmonary vascular resistance as occurs with many of the chronic pulmonary diseases. The interviewer also should collect a detailed list of the patients medications, prescription or otherwise.

Review of Systems

The review of systems is necessary in order to determine if the disease is confined to the respiratory system, or whether the pulmonary complaints are just a manifestation of an illness elsewhere (e.g. conjunctivitis and rhinitis in asthma, sinusitis in bronchiectasis, joint pains, alopecia, depigmentation, and erythema nodosum in sarcoidosis, etc.). Aspiration of postnasal drainage secretions or refluxed gastric contents into the airways at night can cause or exacerbate chronic bronchitis. Unfortunately, this is frequently overlooked as the cause making the airway problem difficult to control.

Occupational History

The patient's occupational history can be very important. Has the patient been in contact with coal, asbestos, or silica? The dust of these materials can lodge in the airways and lungs causing significant disease over time. Other occupational exposures could include molds, pigeons, solvents, paints, etc. *Geographical* history must include travel, immigration, and region of permanent residence. This is especially important if one suspects diseases such as coccidioidomycosis, tuberculosis, or histoplasmosis.

Smoking History

Tobacco smoke inhalation, either primary or secondary, is clearly the leading cause of respiratory disease in adults. The amount of cigarettes smoked usually is recorded by "pack years." This is determined by multiplying the number of packs smoked daily by the years smoked. The more "pack years," the greater the risk of disease.

Family and Social History

The family history includes history of asthma, premature emphysema, chronic bronchitis, cardiac disease, and cystic fibrosis. The social history may identify the excessive use of alcohol. Alcoholism can be associated with periods of loss of consciousness (as in binge drinkers), a decreased efficiency of lung defense mechanisms, with consequent predisposition to aspiration pneumonia as well as bacterial pneumonias of the usual type.

Physical Examination

Physical examination techniques in the assessment of chest disease have been deemphasized since the onset of chest roentgenology. In some instances, roentgenology is much more sensitive than physical examination in detecting disease. This is particularly true for tuberculosis, cystic diseases, carcinoma, nodules, and certain pneumonias. The reverse is often the case, however, with obstructive airway diseases such as acute or chronic bronchitis, early emphysema, and bronchial asthma.

It is our contention that there are certain limitations to the chest film; and all health professionals should become expert in the techniques of physical examination. Physical examination in the pulmonary patient entails the time honored combination of inspection, auscultation, palpation, and percussion.

Inspection

Mastery of the art of inspection may cost a little time, but can be very fruitful. Essentials for proper inspection include a well-lighted, warm room, a patient in the sitting position stripped to the waist (for female patients always prevent embarrassing exposure with adequate draping), a thorough knowledge of the topographic anatomy, and an examiner who is comfortable and not hurried.

Note whether the patient is in pain and if the respirations are noisy or distressed. Identify if the patient is using accessory muscles to breathe. Use of the accessory muscles implies that the work of breathing is increased, as with airways obstruction or reduced lung compliance. Pay careful attention to the skin, breasts, and nutritional state. Some chronic lung diseases result in poor eating habits and malnutrition. Observe the patient for localized areas of bulging or retraction, and the presence of thoracic deformities, such as the increase in the anteroposterior diameter classic in the patient with emphysema (see Fig. 2-1).

Other thoracic deformities of note include pectus carinatum (pigeon breast), characterized by the upper ribs bending inward thrusting the sternum outwards like the keel of a ship (see Fig. 2-2). The "funnel breast" of pectus excavatum (the reverse of carinatum), when severe can diminish vital capacity but usually is a mild asymptomatic congenital defect of cosmetic importance only. The examiner should pay special attention to an exaggerated thoracic and lumbar spinal curvature (kyphosis and scoliosis), as these findings often severely limit lung expansion causing a significant restrictive defect.

Other areas of the body should be carefully inspected. Look at the finger nails and lips to identify if cyanosis (bluish discoloration due to hypoxemia) is present. The digits are also inspected for clubbing (abnormal enlargement of the distal phalanges). Clubbing is a non-specific finding often associated with a chronic decrease in oxygen supply to the tissues (i.e., congenital cyanotic heart disease). The exact mechanism for it remains unknown.

The neck should be inspected for the presence of jugular venous distension (JVD). JVD occurs with right heart failure when pulmonary vascular resistance is chronically elevated. This is common in patients with chronic lung disease that causes hypoxemia.

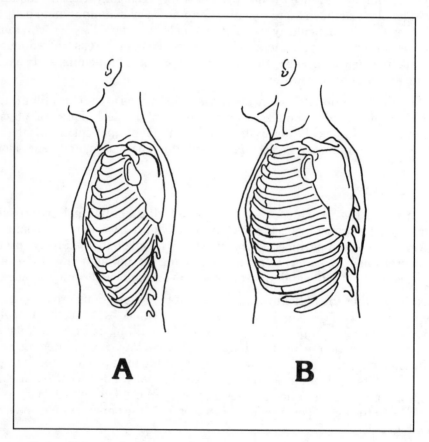

Figure 2-1   A, normal chest configuration; B, increased A-P diameter with hypertrophy of the sternomastoid muscle in the neck typical for patients with chronic obstructive lung disease. (From Dexter, J.R., and Wilkins, R.L.: How to Assess the Patient for Obstructive Lung Disease, 1987 Education Resource Consortium, Claremont, Ca., Vol. 1, #3).

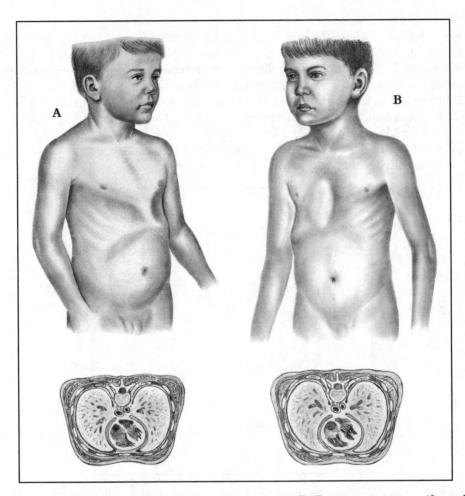

Figure 2-2 A, Pectus carinatum (pigeon chest). B, Pectus excavatum (funnel chest). Deformities of the thorax (From Seidel, H.M., et. al.: Mosby's Guide to Physical Examination, St. Louis, 1987, The C.V. Mosby Co.)

Auscultation

Auscultation, which is the act of listening to sounds produced in the body, has no peer in the evaluation of the state of bronchial patency and the assessment of normal and abnormal breath sounds. Auscultation is performed best with the aid of a stethoscope. The basic stethoscope does not amplify sound but assists in filtering out extraneous noises. Most modern stethoscopes consist of a bell, diaphragm, tubing and ear pieces (see Fig. 2-3). The diaphragm chestpiece is more receptive to high pitched sounds while the bell is best for evaluating low pitched sounds (such as certain heart sounds). The diaphragm is usually better for evaluating normal and abnormal lung sounds.

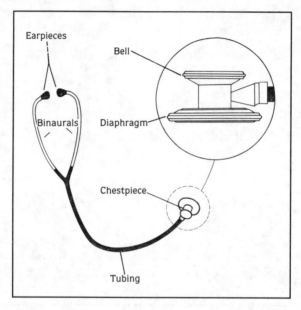

Figure 2-3   Acoustic stethoscope (From Wilkins, R.L., Sheldon, R.L., and Krider, S.J.: Clinical assessment in respiratory care, St. Louis, 1985, The C.V. Mosby Co.)

With the patient in a quiet room, apply the stethoscope firmly against the patient's unclothed chest wall. Application of the stethoscope over clothing should be avoided, since the breath sounds can be significantly altered. Firm pressure is necessary to eliminate chest hair sounds. Instruct the patient to breathe through an open mouth, deeper and faster than normal. Auscultate anteriorly, laterally, and posteriorly in a systematic manner. Listening posteriorly over the lung bases initially may allow detection of abnormal sounds that may clear with several deep breaths. Compare the sounds heard on each side and listen to both inspiration and expiration at each position. To be sure the sounds auscultated are not fictitious, the examiner may instruct the patient to "breath a little deeper" and "faster." Auscultation over the trachea can be particularly helpful in detecting large airway obstruction. Common errors of auscultation that should be avoided are summarized in Table 2-6.

In critically ill patients, the auscultation findings are potentially very important, yet can be difficult to obtain. The patient is often being mechanically ventilated, comatose and bedridden, and unable to cooperate. The examiner should especially make note of the patient's breath sounds in the dependent regions since this is where fluid and mucus will tend to collect initially. To auscultate the dependent regions, the examiner must be more assertive and may need help in turning the patient gently to one side.

Table 2-6.   Errors of Auscultation to Avoid.

Errors	Correct Technique
Listening to breath sounds through the patient's gown	Placing bell or diaphragm directly against the chest wall
Allowing tubing to rub against bed rails or patient's gown	Keeping tubing free from contact with any objects during auscultation
Attempting to auscultate in a noisy room	Turning television or radio off
Interpreting chest hair sounds as adventitious lung sounds	Wetting chest hair before auscultation if thick
Auscultating only the "convenient" areas	Asking alert patient to sit up; rolling comatose patient onto his side to auscultate posterior lobes

Palpation

Palpation also can reveal useful information concerning the thorax and lungs. Palpation of the thorax confirms skeletal abnormalities and identifies localized areas of tenderness in the chest wall. Localized tenderness could indicate rib fractures, costochondritis (inflammation of the cartilage connecting the ribs to the sternum), and other painful rib lesions. One should palpate for masses, pulsations, and areas of crepitation (air trapped in the subcutaneous tissue indicating the presence of subcutaneous emphysema). Subcutaneous air may be present in cases of air leaks caused by severe thoracic injuries, cardiopulmonary resuscitation, insertion of chest tubes and lines and severe asthma attacks.

The greatest value of palpation, however, may be the sensing of transmitted vibrations through the chest wall. This also is known as *fremitus*. The commonly used forms of fremitus in physical diagnosis are vocal and tactile fremitus. This is elicited by having the patient say "ninety-nine," "one-two-three," or "eee-eee-eee." Tactile fremitus is perceived by placing the palmar surfaces of your fingers or the palm itself on the chest wall, overlying the lung. Diminished or absent vocal fremitus suggests inability of the chest wall to register or transmit movements of the tracheo-bronchial air column, e.g., vocal cord failure or airway obstruction. Other conditions leading to reduced vibratory or sound transmission include fluid trapped in the pleural space (pleural effusion) and air in the pleural space (pneumothorax).

Tactile fremitus is increased in conditions that tend to increase the density of the lung. Fremitus is better transmitted through a solid less porous medium such as one would expect in the tissue consolidation of pneumonia. (See Chapter 3 for a complete description of vocal fremitus.)

Pleural friction fremitus is the result of pleurisy as the inflamed pleurae rub against each other. The grating sensation of pleural friction fremitus synchronizes with breathing and may be palpable during both phases.

The neck is palpated to identify if the trachea is in a midline position. The trachea can be deviated to one side due to collapse of an upper lobe, mediastinal tumors, and a large unilateral pleural effusion or pneumothorax.

The peripheral pulses are palpated to detect strength, rhythm, and rate. Weak or absent pulses may indicate poor cardiac function with decreased perfusion. The peripheral pulse may diminish in intensity during inspiration (paradoxical pulse) when severe airways obstruction is present. This is due to the significant drop in pleural pressure that occurs during inspiration in an effort to cause air flow through the obstructed airways. The drop in pleural pressure temporarily reduces blood flow out of the thorax causing the pulse strength to diminish.

The abdomen should be palpated to identify if the liver is enlarged or tender. An enlarged or tender liver is referred to as *hepatomegaly* and is a common finding in patients with right heart failure. A more accurate estimate of the size of the liver can be determined by percussion at the right midclavicular line. Normally, the liver does not span more than 10cm.

Percussion

Percussion of the chest wall can determine the approximate density of the patient's lungs. The popular method of mediate percussion is easily learned, and if performed properly and systematically, is quite helpful in certain situations. This method involves placing the distal phalanx of the middle finger of one hand firmly against the chest wall. This finger should be parallel to the ribs in the intercostal spaces. Strike this finger with a quick, sharp stroke with the middle finger of the other hand (see Fig. 2-4). The resulting sounds are classified as normal resonance, increased resonance, or decreased resonance. Normal resonance has a moderately low pitch with a "drum like" sound. Increased resonance sounds louder and lower in pitch. The opposite of this, decreased resonance, has a high pitched, soft sound of shorter duration.

When percussing the lungs, compare similar positions on both sides of the chest. The decreased resonance of pleural fluid, consolidation, or atelectasis is distinct and therefore more obvious than the increased resonance of emphysema or pneumothorax. Unilateral defects also are easier to identify than bilateral abnormalities since there will be a significant difference in the sounds from one side to the other with unilateral disease.

The magnitude of the diaphragmatic excursion during respiration can be estimated fairly easily by percussion. The lowest margin of resonance is identified with percussion at maximal inspiration and at maximal exhalation. Diaphragm movement is decreased with emphysema and neuromuscular diseases.

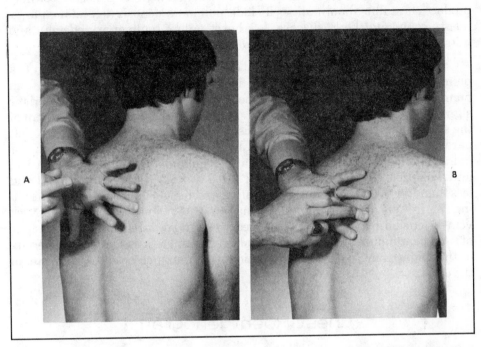

Figure 2-4 Mediate percussion. A, the wrist cocked ready to strike. B, the plexor fingertip is striking the pleximeter finger. Notice that only the pleximeter finger touches the patient's thorax. (From Prior, J.A. and Silberstein, J.S., and Strang, J.M.: Physical diagnosis, ed. 6 St. Louis, 1981, The C.V. Mosby Co.)

Cardiac Examination

The cardiac and respiratory systems are so closely related that a brief discussion of the physical examination and electrocardiographic changes elicited by pulmonary disease is considered important.

The precordium (the chest wall surface overlying the heart) is examined by inspection, palpation, and auscultation. Percussion is of little diagnostic value in most instances. Murmurs, thrills, ventricular lifts (heaves), accentuated heart sounds, ejection clicks, arrhythmias, and friction rubs may be detectable. Murmurs are soft blowing or rasping sounds considered to be an adventitious heart sound. In most cases, a murmur is an indication of abnormal pathology, such as an incompetent valve that causes turbulent blood flow. Abnormal vibrations may be felt over the site of turbulent blood and are referred to as thrills. When the work and forcefulness of the right ventricle is greatly increased, a diffuse lifting impulse is often produced along the lower part of the left sternal border. This is referred to as a lift or heave. A significant increase in pressure in the pulmonary arteries will cause the pulmonic valve to close with more intensity resulting in a louder second heart sound.

Cardiac abnormalities which may be associated with lung diseases or may produce chest film abnormalities include: pulmonic stenosis (left hilar enlargement), congenital heart disease, left heart failure (pulmonary edema), and mitral stenosis (pulmonary hemosiderosis).

Cor pulmonale is the most important example of heart disease secondary to a pulmonary disorder. This ailment is defined as right heart failure resulting from pulmonary hypertension due to pulmonary disease. The most characteristic signs of chronic cor pulmonale are accentuation of the pulmonic component of the second heart sound, jugular venous distension, and the palpation of a left parasternal "slap" during systole. Electrocardiographic changes with cor pulmonale include a tall, peaked P wave (P-pulmonale), right axis deviation, and the ratio of the amplitude of the R and S wave is greater than 1 in V1 and less than 1 in V6. These changes may also be seen in acute cor pulmonale resulting from severe acute bronchial asthma or severe pulmonary embolism. Neck vein distension, hepatomegaly (enlarged liver), and pedal edema are other signs of right heart failure. The heart rate and rhythm are best evaluated by listening in the epigastrium in emphysema patients with an increased A-P diameter of the chest.

Chest Roentgenogram

After interviewing the patient and performing a physical examination, other assessment techniques may be of benefit. The most important of these is the chest roentgenogram. Inspection of a previous chest film is particularly helpful when determining the significance of certain abnormalities, e.g., a solitary nodule. See Fig. 2–5 for a typical P-A chest film. The chest film is especially helpful in detecting changes in lung tissue density as would occur with pneumonia or atelectasis. As lung tissue density increases, the chest film will demonstrate areas of "white-out." With decreases in lung tissue density, the chest film shows darkening of the lung fields.

The basic radiographic evaluation of the lung consists of posteroanterior (P-A) and left lateral views. A variety of supplementary views, including oblique, apical lordotic, expiratory, stereo, decubitus, and prone, may offer additional information. Special procedures such as fluoroscopy, tomography, bronchography, barium swallow, CT scanning, and pulmonary or aortic angiography are invaluable in selected patients.

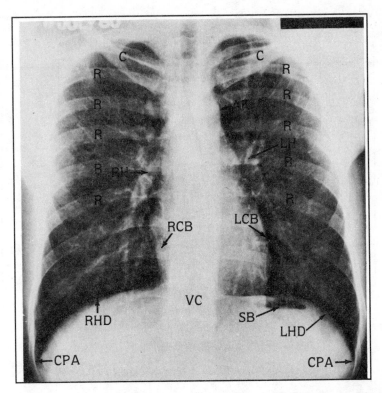

Figure 2-5 Normal posteroanterior chest film, with labeling of important structures. (RHD, right hemidiaphragm; LHD, left hemidiaphragm; CPA, costophrenic angles; RCB, right cardiac border; LCB, left cardiac border; VC, vertebral column; AK, aorticknob; SB, stomach bubble; RH, right hilum; LH, left helium; R, rib; and C, clavicle) (From Wilkins, R.L., Sheldon, R.L., and Krider, S.J.: Clinical assessment in respiratory care, St. Louis, 1985, The C.V. Mosby Co.)

Pulmonary Function Testing

Pulmonary function testing (PFT) has progressed over the last decade from simple spirometry to sophisticated physiologic testing. Few patients can be evaluated completely for pulmonary disease without this modality since it offers several advantages. First, it may uncover a clinically undetectable dysfunction; it can diagnose and characterize the dysfunction; it can objectively measure the severity of disease, and it can monitor the response to therapy.

In the clinical laboratory, complete PFT includes determination of all lung volumes, (see Fig. 2-6) including vital capacity (VC), functional residual capacity (FRC), residual volume (RV), and total lung capacity (TLC), spirometry, diffusing capacity, and often flow-volume loop analysis.

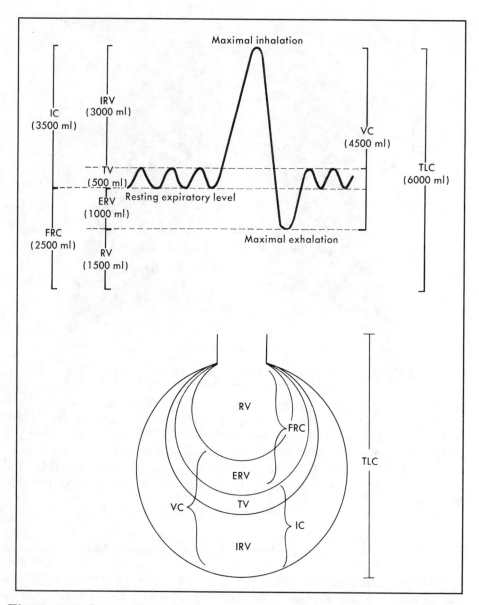

Figure 2-6   Lung volumes and capacities. Representation of a normal spirogram showing the division of lung volumes and capacities. Numbers are for averaged size young adults. (From Spearman, C.B., Sheldon, R.L., and Egan, E.F.: Fundamentals of respiratory therapy, St. Louis, 1982, The C.V. Mosby Co.

Simple spirometry usually provides adequate information. A number of inexpensive electronic and sometimes computerized spirometers capable of accurately measuring such parameters as vital capacity, forced expiratory volume in one second (FEV_1), and peak expiratory flow are available. The information yields reproducible and accurate data. While spirometry alone may not permit specific diagnosis, it can detect obstructive and restrictive disorders and provides an estimate of their severity (see Fig. 2-7).

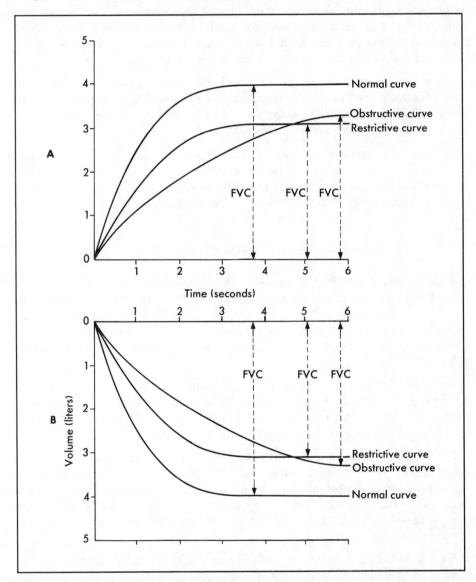

Figure 2-7   Forced vital capacity curves comparing normal, obstructive, and restrictive disorders. A, curves as they appear on commonly available spirometers with tracing beginning at bottom left corner. B, same curves as they appear when tracings begin at upper left corner. (From Spearman, C.B., Sheldon, R.L., and Egan, E.F.: Fundamentals of respiratory therapy, St. Louis, 1982, The C.V. Mosby Co.

In obstructive disorders, spirometry demonstrates a decrease in expiratory flow rates and a normal VC. With more severe obstruction to airflow, the VC may decrease as the result of air trapping. Asthma, chronic bronchitis, and emphysema are the most common obstructive diseases. The response to bronchodilator therapy should be determined in such cases. A 15% increase in the VC or FEV_1 following bronchodilator inhalation is usually considered to represent a significant response to bronchodilator therapy.

In restrictive diseases, spriometry usually demonstrates a decrease in VC and normal flow rates, although occasionally flow rates will be reduced proportional to the reduction in VC. FEV_1 may be reduced in restrictive defects, however the FEV_1/VC is generally normal in such cases.

Spirometry before and after exercise is useful in confirming the diagnosis of exercise induced asthma. In patients undergoing evaluation for possible hypersensitivity airway disease, spirometry after the inhalation of a cholinergic agent or allergenic material may lead to a specific diagnosis.

Arterial Blood Gases

Finally, arterial blood gas analysis (ABG) completes a basic approach to assessment of a typical pulmonary patient. This test is invaluable in evaluating the adequacy of oxygenation and ventilation, and the presence of acid-base disturbances. It is beyond the scope of this chapter to discuss this topic in detail; therefore, our readers are referred to the bibliography for more information if interested.

Simple disturbances of acid-base equilibrium are metabolic and respiratory acidosis and alkalosis. Respiratory acidosis is due to inadequate pulmonary excretion of CO_2 with a resultant increase in PCO_2 (> 45 mmHg). As the PCO_2 elevates, and acidosis occurs, the patient may become lethargic.

Respiratory alkalosis is due to a low PCO_2 (< 35 mmHg) resulting from hyperventilation. Common causes include pain, hypoxia, psychogenic hyperventilation, hypermetabolic states, or excessive ventilation by mechanical ventilators. Respiratory alkalosis frequently is associated with light-headedness, irritability, paraesthesia of the extremities and lips, and possibly even syncope.

Evaluation of the arterial oxygen tension (PaO_2) identifies the ability of the lung to oxygenate the blood. Hypoxemia is generally defined as a PaO_2 below the predicted normal level, and can result from hypoventilation, ventilation/perfusion mismatching, diffusion defect, shunt and high altitude. Hypoxemia is usually the result of a mismatching between ventilation and perfusion in the lung due to pulmonary disease. Evaluation of the arterial PO_2 should always be done with respect to the fraction of inhaled oxygen (FIO_2).

Evaluation of the Neonate

Evaluation of the newborn patient is similar to that of the adult. A careful history, thorough physical examination and use of selected laboratory data is the basis for assessing these patients. While the basic principles remain the same, certain characteristics are uniquely different. Verbal communication with the patient is not possible and cooperation may not be achieved.

History

The newborn's history includes more than just the medical history of the infant. The maternal history is of primary concern. It should provide a description of the mother's health status, detailing any problems that may affect the infant's health status. Of equal importance is the pregnancy history. All illnesses, accidents or drug usage during pregnancy will be described in the pregnancy history. The labor and delivery history describe important facts with regard to labor and method of delivery. Infants born after a long labor are more likely to suffer from asphyxia manifested as hypotension and abnormal heart rates.

The gestational age of the newborn is important to determine since it will influence the incidence of such respiratory diseases as respiratory distress syndrome. Infants born at less than 38 weeks gestation are considered premature.

At the time of delivery, a standard, objective measurement of the newborn's well being is the Apgar score. This is a simple and reliable method of determining the infant's overall health status. It considers five important parameters: heart rate, respiratory effort, muscle tone, reflex irritability, and color. Each of these parameters is evaluated with points of O-2 assigned according to specific physical criteria. The Apgar score is typically recorded at 1 and 5 minutes with higher scores (8-10) indicating better health than lower scores.

Physical Examination

The newborn is carefully inspected for overall color, activity level, body position and level of alertness. Evidence of cyanosis is best identified by inspection of the mucus membranes of the mouth and nail beds in the newborn.

The breathing pattern and effort of breathing should be carefully identified. A common finding with respiratory disease in infants is retractions. Retractions are an inward movement of the chest wall during inspiration. This occurs when the lung compliance is less than that of the chest wall and it may result in intercostal, subcostal, substernal or supraclavicular retractions.

The infant's extremities are palpated for temperature, capillary refill and pulse strength to evaluate cardiac output. Infants with poor perfusion have cool extremities, poor capillary refill and weak or absent pulses.

Initially, auscultation of the infant is best done with the baby resting quietly. For this reason, it may be helpful to auscultate the infant immediately after inspection. Auscultation during episodes of crying does allow assessment of the breath sounds during deeper inspirations. This may result in identification of abnormal sounds that would be missed otherwise. As in the adult, it is important to evaluate lung sounds over the baby's anterior, lateral and posterior chest wall.

Bibliography

Bates, B.: *A Guide to Physical Examination,* 2nd ed., Philadelphia, 1979, J.P. Lippincott Company.

Baum, G.L. and Wolinsky, E.: *Textbook of Pulmonary Diseases,* Boston, 1983, Little, Brown and Company.

Berkow, R.: *The Merck Manual,* New Jersey, 1982, Merck, Sharp & Dohme Research.

Bordow, R.A. and Moser, K.M.: *Manual of Clinical Problems in Pulmonary Medicine,* Boston, 1985, Little, Brown and Company.

Burton, G.G.: *Practical physical diagnosis in respiratory care* in Burton, G.G., Hodgkin, J.E. (eds.): Respiratory Care: A Guide to Clinical Practice, 2nd ed., 1984, J.B. Lippincott, Philadelphia.

Hinshaw, H.C. and Murray, J.F.: *Diseases of the Chest,* Philadelphia, 1980, W.B. Saunders.

Jones, H.B. and Hudson, L.D.: *History and physical examination in Hodgkin,* J.E.; Petty, T.L. (eds.): Chronic Obstructive Pulmonary Disease: Current Concepts, 1987, W.B. Saunders, Philadelphia.

Judge, R.D. and Zuidema, G.D.: *Clinical Diagnosis,* ed. 4, Boston, 1982, Little, Brown and Company.

Lillington, G.A.: *A Diagnostic Approach to Chest Diseases,* ed. 2, Baltimore, 1987, The Williams & Wilkins Co.

Prior, J.A., Silberstein, J.S. and Stang, J.M.: *Physical Diagnosis—The History and Examination of the Patient,* St. Louis, 1981, The C.V. Mosby Company.

Wilkins, R.L., Sheldon, R.L. and Krider, S.J.: *Clinical Assessment in Respiratory Care,* St. Louis, 1985, The C.V. Mosby Company.

CHAPTER
3
Terminology and Mechanisms for Lung Sounds

OBJECTIVES

After reading this chapter, the learner should be able to recognize and describe:

1. The characteristics of the four types of normal breath sounds.

2. The appropriate terms for describing normal and abnormal breath sounds.

3. The proposed mechanism responsible for production of normal breath sounds and possible mechanisms for alteration in the breath sound intensity.

4. Two types of adventitious lung sounds and the appropriate terminology for each.

5. The proposed mechanisms for continuous and discontinuous adventitious lung sounds.

6. The proposed mechanism for a pleural friction rub.

7. Bronchophony, egophony, and whispered pectoriloquy and the significance of each.

Lung sounds can be divided into two major categories: breath sounds and adventitious lung sounds. Breath sounds are normal noises that can be heard on the chest wall with breathing. Adventitious lung sounds are abnormal sounds superimposed on the breath sounds and usually indicate some type of respiratory disorder. First, this chapter will focus on the terminology and mechanisms for breath sounds; a similar review for the adventitious lung sounds and voice sounds will follow.

Breath Sounds

Terminology for Breath Sounds

Normal breath sounds have traditionally been divided into four types: *tracheal, bronchial, bronchovesicular,* and *vesicular.* (See Fig. 3-1 for a diagrammatic representation of these sounds.) Directly over the trachea, the breath sound is particularly loud and high-pitched; it is described as *tracheal.* The tracheal breath sound has a pause between the inspiratory and expiratory components, and the expiratory component is slightly longer. The term *bronchial* is used to describe a similar sound that is also a harsh, high-pitched sound with approximately equal inspiratory and expiratory components. This sound may be heard directly over a major bronchus during normal breathing. Since tracheal and bronchial breath sounds are very similar in characteristics, we prefer use of the term *tracheobronchial* when refering to these loud, tubular type breath sounds. *Bronchovesicular* sounds are a slight variation to the tracheobronchial sound and are heard just distal to the central airways. They are less intense (softer) and lower pitched than bronchial sounds but maintain an equal inspiratory and expiratory component (See Fig. 3-1). The *vesicular* breath sound is significantly softer in intensity and primarily is an inspiratory sound. The expiratory component of the vesicular breath sound is normally minimal, only occurring during the initial one third of the expiratory phase. It is normally heard over all areas of the chest distal to the central airways (See Fig. 3-2).

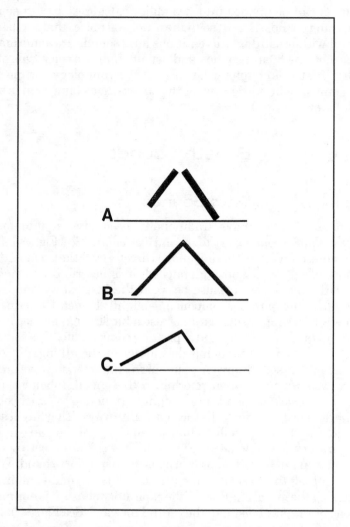

Figure 3-1 Diagrams for Normal Breath Sounds; A—tracheobronchial, B—bronchovesicular, C—vesicular. Upstroke represents inspiration and downstroke represents expiration. The thickness of the line indicates sound intensity.

The term "vesicular" is derived from the Latin word for small vessels and originated back when clinicians thought this sound resulted from air entry into the small vessels (alveoli). We now know, however, that the peripheral lung units in healthy individuals are essentially silent.

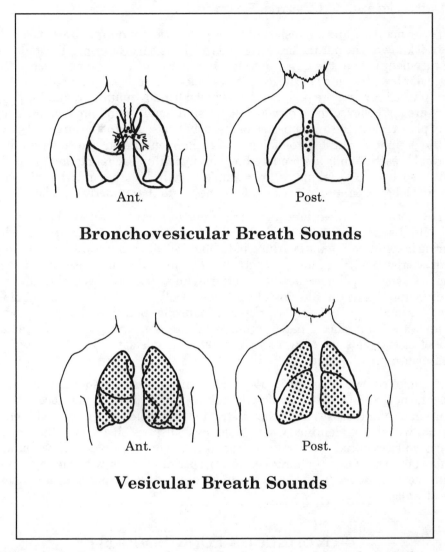

Figure 3-2 Location on chest wall where normal bronchovesicular and vesicular type breath sounds are heard.

When vesicular breath sounds are found to be of less intensity than expected, they are described as *diminished (reduced)* or even *absent* in extreme cases. If the peripheral breath sound increases in intensity, it is described as *harsh;* if it also takes on a more prominent expiratory component it is described as *tracheobronchial* (tubular).

Mechanisms of Breath Sounds

The exact mechanisms responsible for production of normal breath sounds are not known. The normal breath sounds are believed to be primarily produced by turbulent flow in the larger airways; however, the inspiratory phase of the vesicular breath sound is believed to be produced more distally than the expiratory phase.[1] Since more peripheral airways normally maintain laminar flow, they are not believed to be responsible for significant sound production. They may play a role in the transmission of the turbulent sounds of the larger airways to the peripheral chest. The majority of experimental evidence suggests that normal breath sounds are produced regionally within each lung and probably within each lobe.[2] This implies, for example, that the breath sounds heard over a specific lobe probably are a result of air entry into that underlying lobe.

The normal air-filled lung acts as a filter to sound. It alters the tracheobronchial sounds of the central airways to a softer version heard primarily during inspiration. Changes in lung pathology will alter the sound transmission characteristics of the lung parenchyma. Diseases that increase lung tissue density usually will increase the sound transmission qualities and result in a significant loss in the filtering effect. As a result, tracheobronchial (tubular) breath sounds may be heard over areas of consolidation, e.g. lobar pneumonia or atelectasis, provided a patent bronchus is present. An obstructed bronchus will block transmission of the bronchial sounds and lead to absent or markedly diminished breath sounds.

Diminished breath sounds may result from decreases in sound generation (less turbulent flow) with shallow breathing patterns. This may occur with neuromuscular diseases and other restrictive lung defects. Diminished breath sounds will also be identified when the sound transmission ability of the lung or chest wall is reduced and results in more filtering of the turbulent flow sounds. This can occur when the lung becomes hyperinflated (as with emphysema), with pleural disease (effusion or pneumothorax), or with muscular and obese chest walls.

Adventitious Lung Sounds

Terminology for Adventitious Lung Sounds

Based on acoustical recordings and analysis of lung sounds, the adventitious sounds can be divided into two categories: continuous and discontinuous. Continuous lung sounds are musical sounds with a constant pitch. Their duration may extend from very short (200 msec) to several seconds. They are more often heard during exhalation and are associated with obstruction of airways. Discontinuous adventitious lung sounds are intermittent, crackling or bubbling sounds of short duration (< 20 msec). These brief bursts of sound are heard most commonly during inspiration and may be present with both restrictive and obstructive defects (See Fig. 3–3).

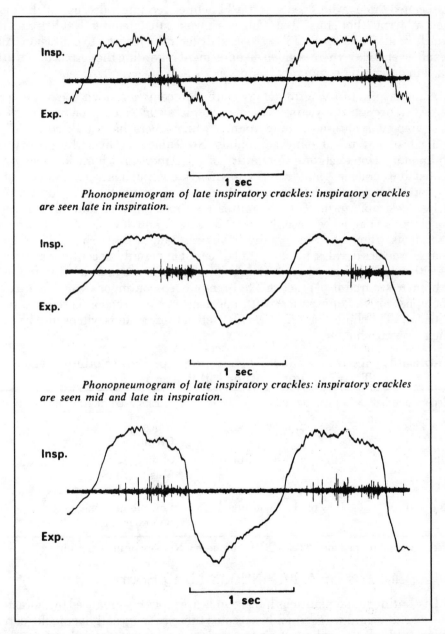

Phonopneumogram of late inspiratory crackles: inspiratory crackles are seen late in inspiration.

Phonopneumogram of late inspiratory crackles: inspiratory crackles are seen mid and late in inspiration.

Figure 3-3   Phonopneumograms illustrating inspiratory crackles heard late (A) mid and late, (B) and throughout, (C) inspiration. (From Nath, A.R., and Capel, L.H.: Inspiratory crackles early and late. Thorax 29:223, 1974.)

The terms used to describe the adventitious lung sounds lack standardization even today.[3] Originally Laennec used the term "rale" for all abnormal sounds with four subgroups: moist, mucous, sonorous, and sibilant.[4] When patients associated "rale" with "death rattle," Laennec recommended use of the more neutral term "rhonchus." Later his work was translated into English and the words "rales" and "rhonchi" were used differently, leading to confusion. As a result, even today, there is much disagreement regarding the correct terms to be used in describing commonly heard sounds.

A major part of the terminology confusion centers around use of the term "rale."[5] Through the years, some experts have suggested it be used only for describing discontinuous lung sounds while others have utilized "rale" to indicate other types of abnormal sounds. (See Table 3–1) Given this history, the Pulmonary Nomenclature Committee of the American Thoracic Society has stated that "crackles" and "rales" are synonymous, but has recommended use of the term "crackles" to describe discontinuous sounds and has labeled "rales" as a less desirable term. The committee also recommends that high-pitched, continuous sounds be described as "wheezes" and low-pitched, continuous sounds as "rhonchi." Since many have been taught that "rhonchi" refers to coarse crackles or rales, there might be benefit in describing continuous sounds as either low-pitched wheezes or high-pitched wheezes and deleting the term "rhonchi" from clinical practice. The high-pitched, continuous sound heard over the upper airway of a patient with upper airway obstruction is referred to as "stridor." The clinical significance for each of these sounds will be discussed in the following chapter.

Table 3-1. Recommended* Terminology for Lung Sounds Versus Terminology in other Publications

Recommended	Classification	Terms used in other publications
Crackles	Discontinuous	Rales Crepitations
Wheezes	High-pitched, continuous	Sibilant rales Musical rales Sibilant rhonchus
Rhonchi	Low-pitched, continuous	Low-pitched wheeze Sonorous rales

*Recommendations from ATS-ACCP Pulmonary Nomenclature Committee.

Mechanisms of Adventitious Lung Sounds

Discontinuous adventitious lung sounds are probably produced by more than one mechanism. Two commonly accepted theories suggest that crackles can be produced by the bubbling of air through airway secretions or by the sudden opening of small airways. Crackles associated with the movement of airway secretions in larger airways are typically coarse and may occur during both inspiration and expiration. They may clear if the patient coughs effectively or with suctioning.

Crackles associated with the sudden opening of airways may be produced by a rapid equalization of pressure between patent and collapsed airways.[6,7] These crackles are inspiratory sounds, which may occur when peripheral airways pop open as collapsed (atelectatic) regions are inflated (see Fig. 3-4). With atelectasis due to a shallow breathing pattern, the crackles often disappear after a few deep breaths or after changes in position, whereas with pulmonary fibrosis, the crackles persist. In mild pulmonary fibrosis, the crackles are predominantly heard late in inspiration, but may become pan-inspiratory with an end-inspiratory accentuation as the disease progresses. Late-inspiratory crackles are often repetitive with several respiratory cycles and initially identified in dependent lung zones. Late-inspiratory crackles are very suggestive of a restrictive lung defect and indicate a loss in lung volume.

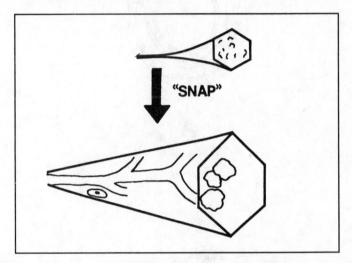

"SNAP"

Figure 3-4   Sudden re-expansion of collapsed peripheral airways. (From Murphy, R.L.H.: Lung sounds. Basics of Respiratory Disease, Vol. 8, #4, Am Thor Soc, 1980.)

More proximal airways may collapse during exhalation when bronchial wall compliance increases. During the subsequent inspiration, the airways will pop open intermittently and produce different inspiratory crackles. In such cases, the crackles primarily occur early in inspiration and may not be affected by coughing or changes in position. Early-inspiratory crackles are scanty, low-pitched and audible at the mouth as well as over the chest. They could be suggestive of chronic obstructive airway diseases that affect bronchial wall compliance.[8]

Continuous adventitious lung sounds are believed to result from airway narrowing, which initially causes rapid airflow past the site of obstruction[9] (see Fig. 3-5). The more rapid airflow decreases lateral airway wall pressures, and results in the opposite walls pulling closer together and briefly touching. As a result, flow is briefly interrupted and airway pressure increases. The airway now returns to a more open position permitting airflow to return (see Fig. 3-6). The cycle repeats itself rapidly causing vibration of airway walls. This process will continue until insufficient flow occurs as when the patient tires or until the airway obstruction is relieved.

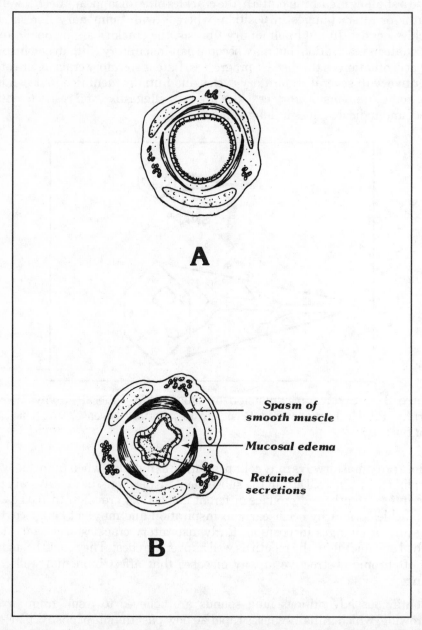

Figure 3-5 A, normal airway. B, obstructed airway, with bronchospasm, musocal edema and airway secretions contributing to the reduction in airway lumen. (From Wilkins, R.L., and Dexter, J.: How to Assess the Patient for Obstructive Lung Disease, Education Resource Consortium, Claremont, Ca. Vol. 1, #3, 1987.)

The pitch of the continuous adventitious sound is determined by the relationship between flowrate and degree of obstruction. More rapid flows or tighter obstruction result in higher pitched sounds. Lower flowrates or less obstruction will result in lower pitched sounds.

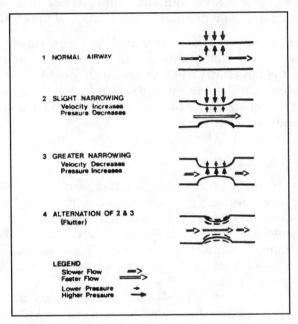

Figure 3-6 Proposed mechanism for production of continuous type of adventitious lung sound. The stability of the airway wall depends upon a balance between internal air pressure and external forces (1). When narrowing of the lumen occurs, the air velocity must increase to maintain a constant mass flow rate (2). This leads to a decrease in pressure in the constricted area, thus allowing external forces to further collapse the airway (3). When the lumen has been reduced so much that the flow rate decreases, the process begins to reverse itself as the pressure inside the airway increases and reopens the lumen. (From Murphy, R.L.H.: Lung sounds. Basics of Respiratory Disease, Vol. 8, #4, Am Thor Soc, 1980.)

During expiration, bronchi become progressively smaller. This is accentuated when intrathoracic pressures increase during forced breathing as when the patient actively forces the air out of his chest. As a result, the process of producing continuous adventitious lung sounds is likely to occur more frequently and for longer periods during expiration. The opposite is true during inspiration when intrathoracic airways are less narrow. A variable obstruction of extrathoracic airways (trachea, larynx) will result more often in continuous adventitious lung sounds during inspiration. This occurs since airway pressure distal to the obstruction is decreased significantly in relation to atmospheric pressure outside the airway during inspiration. This pressure gradient narrows the site of obstruction further and sets up the situation needed to produce inspiratory stridor or wheezes. During expiration, a rising airway pressure produces a pressure gradient that is positive from inside to outside the airway and the obstruction lessens. Thus, extrathoracic airway obstruction is less likely to result in continuous adventitious lung sounds during expiration. If the obstruction becomes fixed or severe enough, the sound "stridor" will be heard during inspiration and expiration regardless of the location of the obstruction.

It is important to note that only the larger bronchi are capable of generating continuous adventitious lung sounds. Small airways have significantly lower flowrates than the larger airways and are much less likely to be a source of expiratory wheezes. Only two or three peripheral generations of bronchial airways past the segmental bronchi are believed to be capable of producing continuous sounds.

Qualifying Adjectives

The terms used to qualify the adventitious lung sounds also lack standardization. Experts now suggest using adjectives that have a scientific basis consistent with waveform analysis of the acoustical characteristics. Terms such as "wet," "dry," "sonorous," and "sibilant," which have no logical basis, should be replaced with more accurate terms such as "high-pitched," "low-pitched," "fine," "medium" and "coarse." We will use the terms "fine," "medium," and "coarse" to indicate the pitch of discontinuous abnormal lung sounds. For example, "fine crackles" would imply high-pitched sounds and "coarse crackles" would imply "low-pitched sounds." We will use "mild," "moderate," and "severe" to indicate the intensity of continuous abnormal lung sounds such as wheezes.

A more important description of diagnostic value is the timing of the adventitious sounds during the respiratory cycle. Abnormal sounds should be described as "inspiratory'," "expiratory'," or both. In addition, the specific timing during inspiration (i.e., late-inspiratory crackles) may be of some help. The clinical significance of such descriptions is described more extensively in the next chapter.

Pleural Friction Rub

Normally, the smooth, moist layers of the pleura slide silently on one another during breathing. Alterations in the pleura from inflammation or fibrin deposits can result in added friction between the pleural layers. The sound produced is usually non-musical and has been compared to the creaking sound of old leather. Friction rubs are usually lower pitched, of longer duration than pulmonary crackles, and commonly are present during both inspiration and expiration; however, they may be mistaken for sounds emanating from within the lung.

Voice Sounds

Vocal resonance is created as the vibrations of phonation travel down the tracheobronchial tree and throughout the lung parenchyma. A normal air-filled lung transmits low frequency sounds (< 200 Hz) but higher frequencies are selectively filtered and attenuated. As a result, speech heard through a stethoscope over normal lung is heard as a low-pitched mumble. Alteration in lung pathology will change the transmission of voice sounds, resulting in either increased or decreased transmission of vocal resonance.

An increase in vocal resonance, known as *bronchophony,* results in louder and clearer voice sounds over the affected area. This occurs with increases in lung tissue density, as in lung consolidation from pneumonia or atelectasis. In such cases, the acoustical filtering ability of the lung is reduced. Bronchophony is easier to detect when it is unilateral and associated with bronchial breath sounds.

A reduction in vocal resonance occurs when lung tissue density decreases, resulting in more filtering of sound. This typically is identified with pulmonary hyperinflation disorders such as emphysema and acute asthma and is bilateral in such cases. Decreased vocal resonance also is noted over areas of the lung separated from the chest wall by pneumothorax or pleural effusion.

When the voice sound increases in intensity and takes on a nasal or "bleating" quality, it is described as *egophony.* Egophony generally is identified over areas of the chest where bronchophony is present. The exact reason for this change in the voice sound is unknown. It is identified by asking the patient to say "e-e-e." If egophony is present, the "e-e-e" will be heard as "a-a-a" over the peripheral chest wall with a stethoscope. This most frequently is identified over consolidated lung, such as over an area of lobar pneumonia or an area of compressed lung above a pleural effusion.

Whispering creates high-frequency vibrations that are filtered out selectively by normal lung tissue and normally heard as muffled, low-pitched sounds over the chest wall. When consolidation is present, however, the lung loses its selective transmitter quality, and the whispering is transmitted to the chest wall with more clarity. This sign, known as *whispered pectoriloquy,* is especially helpful to identify in patients with small or patchy areas of lung consolidation where more obvious signs may be absent. It is usually elicited by having the patient whisper 1-2-3 or 99.

Miscellaneous Sounds

In patients with chest hair, a crackling noise may be heard from the chest hair rubbing on the diaphragm of the stethoscope. Firm pressure of the stethoscope on the skin, or wetting the hair, will help to eliminate this extraneous sound. When air is present in the subcutaneous tissue (subcutaneous emphysema), a crackling noise can be heard when the stethoscope is pressed down over the affected area. When air is present in the mediastinum (pneumo-mediastinum) and sometimes with a left pneumothorax, a crunching or crackling sound may be heard with each heart beat, and is referred to as a *systolic or xiphisternal crunch* . If the patient has fractured ribs or a fractured sternum, the ends of the bone may rub against one another and cause a clicking sound. This is referred to as *bone crepitus*. If water is present in the tubing between a mechanical ventilator and an endotracheal or tracheostomy tube, a gurgling or bubbling sound might be confused with coarse rales when listening over the chest with a stethoscope. With some PEEP (positive end-expiratory pressure) systems on ventilators, a continuous high-pitched expiratory sound which might be confused with a wheeze, is sometimes heard. It is important to identify the proper source of these sounds, rather than mistaking them as arising from within the lungs.

Summary

Normal breath sounds can be categorized into three general types: tracheobronchial, bronchovesicular, and vesicular. There is no uniform agreement as to the origin of breath sounds, but most feel that inspiratory sounds are produced in the lung, (not in the upper airways or the alveoli, but somewhere in between) while the expiratory phase is produced more centrally.

When the vesicular breath sound increases in intensity, it is described as harsh, tubular, or tracheobronchial. This occurs when the filtering properties of the lung parenchyma are reduced with consolidation. Diminished breath sounds result when the filtering effect of the lung is increased, as with emphysema. A hyperinflated lung transmits sound frequencies poorly.

Adventitious lung sounds are abnormal sounds superimposed on the breath sounds. They are divided into continuous and discontinuous types. Continuous adventitious lung sounds are most often the result of airways obstruction that causes rapid airflow through the obstructed site with resulting airway wall vibration. It has been recommended that they be called "wheezes" if high-pitched and "rhonchi" if low-pitched. There might be benefit, however, in eliminating the terms "rhonchus" or "rhonchi" and simply describing this sound as a low-pitched "wheeze." "Stridor" is also a continuous type of abnormal sound produced by obstruction of the upper airway.

Discontinuous adventitious lung sounds are produced by the sudden opening of collapsed airways or by the movement of air through excessive airway secretions. While most clinicians refer to these sounds as "rales," some experts prefer use of the term "crackles." These sounds are present predominantly during the inspiratory phase, while continuous sounds, (e.g., wheezes), are heard more commonly during exhalation.

References

1. Loudon, R, and Murphy, RLH: *Lung sounds,* Am Rev Respir Dis 130:663-673, 1984.

2. Kraman, SS: *Vesicular (normal) lung sounds: How are they made, where do they come from, and what do they mean?* Sem in Resp Med 6:183, 1985.

3. Pasterkamp, H, Montgomery, M, and Wiebicke, W: *Nomenclature used by health care professionals to describe breath sounds in asthma,* Chest 92: 346, 1987.

4. Andrews, JL and Badger, TL: *Lung sounds through the ages,* JAMA 241:2625, 1979.

5. Wilkins, RL, Dexter, JR, and Smith, JR: *Survey of adventitious lung sound terminology in case reports,* Chest 85:523, 1984.

6. Polysongsang, Y and Schonfeld, SA: *Mechanism of production of crackles after atelectasis during low-volume breathing,* Am Rev Resp Dis 126:413, 1982.

7. Forgacs, P: *The functional basis of pulmonary sounds,* Chest 73:399, 1978.

8. Nath, AR and Capel, LH: *Inspiratory crackles—early and late,* Thorax 29:223, 1974.

9. Waring, WW, Beckerman, RC, and Hopkins, RL: Continuous adventitious lung sounds: *Site and method of production and significance,* Sem in Resp Med 6:201, 1985.

Suggested Reading

Cugell, DW: *Lung sounds: Classification and controversies,* Sem in Resp Med 6:180, 1985.

Forgacs, P: *Lung Sounds,* Bailliere Tindall, London, 1978.

Murphy, RLH: *Discontinuous adventitious lung sounds,* Sem in Resp Med 6:210, 1985.

Murphy, RLH and Holford, SK: *Lung Sounds,* Basics of RD 8:1-6, 1980.

Robertson, JA and Coope, R: *Rales, rhonchi and Laennec.* Lancet 2:417, 1957.

Report of the ATS-ACCP Ad Hoc Subcommittee on Pulmonary Nomenclature. Am Thor Soc News, 1977, Vol. 3, p. 51.

CHAPTER
4
Clinical Applications of
Lung Sounds

Objectives:

After reading this chapter, the learner should be able to recognize and describe:

1. The significance of normal breath sound intensity at any chest wall location and potential causes for reduction in intensity.

2. The relationship between breath sound intensity and the degree of chronic obstructive lung disease.

3. Why it is important to assess the expiratory component of the vesicular breath sound and the significance of changes in it.

4. The therapy that may be indicated by decreased breath sounds, bronchial breath sounds, late-inspiratory or coarse crackles, wheezes, and stridor.

5. The characteristics of wheezing that should be evaluated and how these characteristics change with alteration in the degree of airways obstruction.

6. Why auscultation may be of less value in the neonate than the adult.

7. Auscultation and other physical findings typical for: atelectasis, pneumonia, congestive heart failure, pleural effusion, pulmonary fibrosis, pneumothorax, asthma, chronic bronchitis, and emphysema.

This chapter will review normal and abnormal lung sounds in the light of what they tell us about the status of the lungs. Specifically, chest auscultation can assist in making the initial assessment and help identify what other diagnostic techniques may or may not be needed. In addition, lung sounds can be very helpful in evaluating the effects of treatment on the pulmonary system. A better understanding of this information should allow clinicians to provide more appropriate and cost-effective health care.

Breath Sounds

Vesicular Breath Sounds

An important aspect of auscultation is the process of identifying the intensity (loudness) of the vesicular breath sound. This requires that clinicians have an appreciation for the expected normal breath sound intensity (BSI). Through experience, the ability to recognize slight abnormalities in BSI becomes easier. Comparing one side to another is helpful in recognizing unilateral defects. This has limitations, however, since research has recently shown that normal individuals may have slight variations in BSI at similar locations in opposite lungs.[1]

Normal breath sound intensity at a single location on the chest wall correlates with the degree of ventilation in the underlying lobe. A normal BSI in the adult implies that underlying regional ventilation is occurring, but the exact degree cannot be determined. A decrease in BSI may be the result of diminished ventilation in the underlying lobe, poor sound transmission qualities of the lung, or both. Diminished regional ventilation may occur with bronchial intubation, mucus plugging, lung consolidation, or bronchial obstruction. Poor sound transmission qualities of the lung occur with hyperinflation, as in acute or chronic airways obstruction.

In cases of airways obstruction, decreased ventilation and sound transmission contribute to diminished BSI. Therapy such as postural drainage, bronchial hygiene techniques, and bronchodilators may result in better regional ventilation and BSI in affected areas. Therapy that results in a reversal of airway(s) obstruction and diminished hyperinflation should result in a more normal BSI. This improvement is more likely to occur in asthma than emphysema since airway obstruction is due to more reversible changes in the lung with asthma.

Evaluating the BSI over multiple sites on the chest wall can help determine the degree of chronic airflow obstruction. Studies have shown a good correlation between BSI scores and expiratory flowrate parameters from spirograms.[2-4] This requires estimating the BSI on a scale of 0 - 3 with 0 = absent, 1 = diminished, 2 = normal and 3 = louder than expected normal. This examination is made at six locations on the chest wall; bilaterally over the upper anterior regions, in the mid-axillae, and at the posterior bases. BSI scores then are tabulated and correlated with pulmonary function results.

Results have shown that normal BSI scores nearly always ruled out the presence of severe airways obstruction. Definitely reduced BSI scores were strong indications of severe airways obstruction. Mild obstructive defects are not quantified easily with this method since patients with moderate reduction in BSI scores had a variety of pulmonary function results.

These results suggest that when the history or physical examination imply chronic airways obstruction, careful evaluation of the breath sounds may help quantify the degree of obstruction present. Pre-op patients with mild to severe reductions in BSI scores should have spirograms to evaluate further the pulmonary system and its ability to tolerate the planned surgery.

Tracheobronchial Breath Sounds

Evaluating the expiratory component of the vesicular breath sound is important. Normally it is faint and heard only during the early part of exhalation. For this reason it is often ignored. One of the first signs of lung congestion is a change in the vesicular breath sound to more of a tracheobronchial sound. In such cases the breath sound increases in pitch and intensity and the expiratory component of the breath sound becomes more prominent. This change is subtle and often missed. It occurs initially in the dependent regions of the lungs in the bed-ridden patient. Since these areas on the chest wall are difficult to assess, especially in the comatose patient, this abnormality often is not detected until more obvious abnormalities are present.

When tracheobronchial type breath sounds are detected over the lung fields, lung expansion therapies and/or postural drainage may be indicated. If the therapy results in re-expansion of the atelectatic regions, the breath sound should return to more of a vesicular type.

While the chest roentgenogram has become the cornerstone of chest assessment, its diagnostic yield is low in many cases. Evaluating the breath sounds may, in some cases, allow omission of a routine chest roentgenogram. Normal breath sounds in patients with respiratory complaints or fever ruled out pneumonia with greater than 95% certainty in one study.[5] This suggests that careful attention to the patient's breath sounds may allow for a reduction in unnecessary radiation exposure and costs to the patient.

Adventitious Lung Sounds

Crackles

An important aspect of crackles (also known as rales) to evaluate is their timing during the respiratory cycle. Diffuse pan-inspiratory or late-inspiratory crackles are highly suggestive of a restrictive lung defect. This may occur with asbestosis, atelectasis, pulmonary fibrosis, congestive heart failure (CHF), or pneumonia. The late-inspiratory crackles usually are superimposed on a harsh or bronchial breath sound. With atelectasis, the crackles tend to be gravity dependent, and commonly clear with several deep breaths, changes in position, or coughing.

Patients with interstitial pneumonia or fibrosis typically have "fine" or "dry" inspiratory crackles (see Fig. 4-1). They appear to be related to the severity of the illness. In early stages, the crackles may be heard only in the bases but progress to the upper lobes with advancing disease.

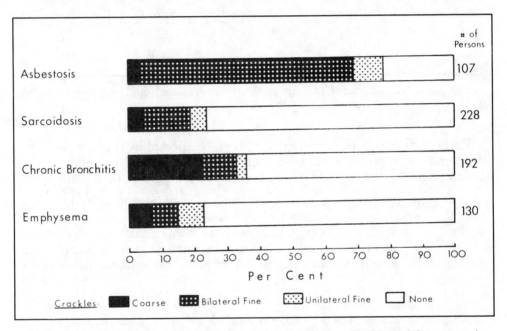

Figure 4-1   Incidence and types of crackles according to clinical diagnoses in 657 patients. (From Epler, G.R., Carrington, C.B. and Gaensler, E.A.: Crackles (rales) in the interstitial pulmonary diseases. Chest 73:333, 1978.)

Late-inspiratory crackles may be reversible in certain clinical conditions such as atelectasis, pneumonia and CHF. Therapy that reexpands atelectatic regions, such as IPPB, incentive spirometry and turning the patient should help resolve the crackles in these situations. In CHF patients, diuretics also may help. With pulmonary fibrosis, the inspiratory crackles persist in spite of deep breaths since they are a result of permanent pathologic changes in the lung.

In patients with chronic obstructive pulmonary disease (COPD), early inspiratory crackles may be identified. In such cases the crackles are scanty and often radiate to the mouth. They are not affected by coughing or changes in position. Their presence may indicate that more severe obstructive disease is present.

Nath and Capel[6] demonstrated that in a group of patients with obstructive lung disease, those with early-inspiratory crackles had lower expiratory flows on the average (lower FEV_1/FVC ratios) than those without early-inspiratory crackles (see Table 4-1). This implies that early-inspiratory crackles are a sign of more significant chronic airflow obstruction in patients with obstructive lung disease.

Table 4-1. FEV_1/FVC% in 56 Patients with Early and Late Inspiratory Crackles.*

Inspiratory Crackles	No. of Patients	FEV_1/FVC		
		Mean %	Range	SD
Early	24	31	19-39	5.6
Late	32	74	58-90	9.5

*From Nath, A.R., and Capel, L.H.: Inspiratory crackles—early and late. Thorax 29:223, 1974.

Early inspiratory crackles are not likely to be affected by therapy since the mechanisms responsible for them (altered bronchial wall compliance and elastic recoil) are the result of more permanent alterations in lung pathology.

Coarse, gurgling crackles indicate excessive airway secretions. In this situation, the crackles tend to occur in both inhalation and exhalation as air moves across the secretions. Gurgling crackles usually will clear with an effective cough or with tracheal suctioning. They are most often present in patients with a diminished cough due to artificial airways, neuromuscular diseases, or medications.

Coarse inspiratory crackles are a common finding in bronchiectasis. The crackles of bronchiectasis typically are located early to mid-inspiration and are more profuse than in chronic bronchitis and emphysema.[7] They tend to become less in number after coughing.

Inspiratory crackles are generally considered an abnormality, but may be identified in patients with normal lungs in certain situations. Profuse inspiratory crackles have been identified in normal subjects during inhalation following a maximal exhalation.[8] They are rarely identified during breathing from resting lung volume in normal individuals. Therefore, inspiratory crackles should be considered an abnormality only when they occur during inspiration from a resting lung volume.

Wheezes

When wheezing is noted during auscultation, several characteristics should be identified. Wheezes may be classified as high or low pitched, inspiratory or expiratory, short or long and single or multiple. Identifying these characteristics will help determine the severity and location of the airway(s) obstruction and the response to therapy. Changes in these characteristics may be subtle and go unnoticed if auscultation is done too rapidly.

The pitch of the wheeze is a function of the relationship between the degree of airways obstruction and the flowrate of air past the obstruction. In the patient with good respiratory effort, the pitch of the wheeze increases as the airways obstruction worsens. If the patient tires and respiratory effort is diminished, tighter airways obstruction may result in lower inspiratory and expiratory flowrates and lower pitched wheezes or none at all. The intensity of the sound also will be decreased in such cases.

Baughman and Loudon[9] have documented that improvements in expiratory flowrates (FEV_1) in asthmatics treated with bronchodilators are associated with a reduction in the sound frequency of the wheeze. Hence, bronchodilator therapy may lower the pitch of the wheeze if it is effective. Other clinical parameters such as the vital signs will help confirm that the reduction in pitch is the result of bronchodilation and not respiratory failure.

The timing of the wheeze during the respiratory cycle may provide clues as to the location and severity of obstruction. As mentioned in Chapter 3, inspiratory wheezing more frequently is associated with extrathoracic lesions such as laryngeal narrowing from a tumor or vocal cord paralysis, and expiratory wheezing is more frequently associated with intrathoracic lesions such as a cylindroma neoplasm in the lower trachea. Exceptions do occur. A bronchial tumor or foreign body aspiration that produces a fixed airway obstruction typically results in both inspiratory and expiratory wheezing. It is not uncommon for patients with chronic bronchitis, bronchiectasis, or cystic fibrosis to have both inspiratory and expiratory wheezes. Inspiratory wheezes may be heard following a series of crackles in fibrosing lung diseases. The wheezing in this situation usually occurs late in inspiration.

Studies have documented a relationship between the proportion of the respiratory cycle occupied by wheezing and flowrate parameters.[9, 10] Asthmatic patients were treated with bronchodilators; and as expiratory flowrate parameters improved, the proportion of the respiratory cycle in which wheezing occurred was reduced (see Fig. 4–2 and 4–3). For example, wheezing may be heard during both inspiration and expiration or be pan-expiratory before treatment. After treatment, if obstruction is improved, the wheezing may be heard only during the last half of expiration, occupying a shorter portion of the respiratory cycle. Precise evaluation of changes in wheezing duration is not possible without phonopneumography but extremes are recognized easily with auscultation.

Since each wheeze indicates partial obstruction of a bronchus, the number of wheezes helps assess the extent of disease. Single (or localized) wheezes indicate a localized area of narrowing while multiple (generalized) wheezes indicate more widespread disorders such as asthma or bronchitis.

Identifying the anatomical position where wheezing is loudest will also help indicate the origin. Wheezing that transmits to the mouth generally indicates

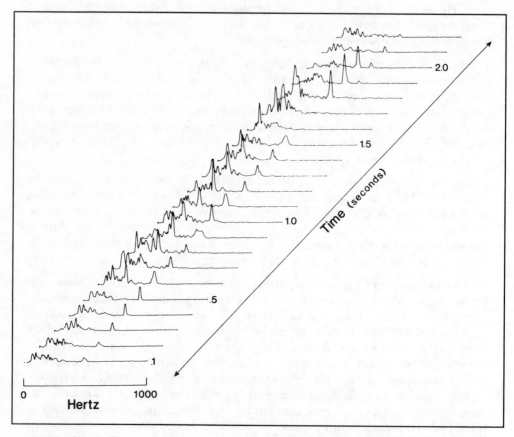

Figure 4-2 Complex set of wheezes in asthmatic with acute bronchospasm. Line 1 represents beginning of expiration. Wheezing was heard on inspiration and expiration, and several peaks are identified, even at same moment in breath cycle (polyphonia). This patient has wheezing in 19 or 22 segments making up her breath cycle. Her Tw/Ttot (wheezing time of total cycle) = 1.9 secs/2.2 secs = 0.86. Highest pitch of any wheeze is 500 Hz.

that larger airways are involved, whereas wheezing heard only over the peripheral chest is probably the result of obstruction in more peripheral airways.

Evaluating the sounds heard over the trachea can be of value in assessment of asthmatic patients. Husodo,[11] in a study of 181 wheezing patients, identified that the wheezing could be heard only over the trachea in 41 (23%) of the patients. Thus, had tracheal auscultation not been done, the wheezes would have been missed in numerous patients. Perhaps transmission of the sounds is affected by flow direction within the airway and are convected towards the upper airway during exhalation. When wheezing is heard only over the larynx or trachea, one should consider the possibility of large airway obstruction.

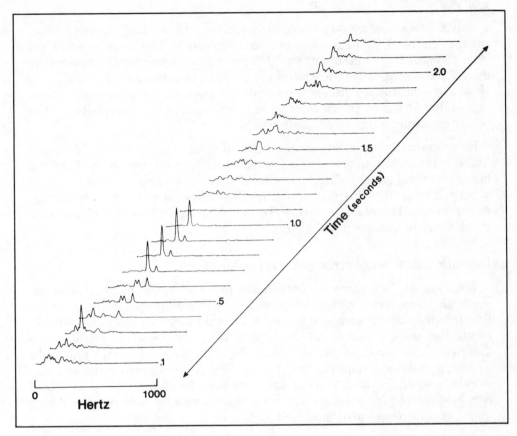

Figure 4-3 Same patient as in Figure 4-2 after bronchodilators. Line 1 marks beginning of expiration. Time of wheezing is now 0.8 secs of a total of 2.6 secs (Tw/Ttot - 0.31). Highest frequency is now 300 Hz. (From Baughman, R.P., and Loudon, R.G.: Quantification of wheezing in acute asthma. Chest 86:718, 1984.)

Monophonic Wheezing

A monophonic wheeze is a single musical note. This musical note is the result of a single bronchus narrowed to nearly complete closure. The sound may be heard throughout the respiratory cycle if the stenosis is rigid. If the obstruction is variable as the flexible bronchus alters position with breathing, the wheeze may be heard only during a portion of the respiratory cycle.

Monophonic wheezes may be single or multiple and are a characteristic sign of asthma. In patients with multiple monophonic wheezes, individual notes often begin and end at different times but overlap. The illusion that many wheezes are being heard is due to the wide transmission of a few loud notes to most areas of the chest wall.

Polyphonic Wheezing

Polyphonic wheezing is confined to expiration and consists of several different musical notes that start and end simultaneously. The sound created has been compared to a dissonant chord. This type of wheezing is produced by dynamic compression of the central bronchi and is a common sign of chronic obstructive pulmonary disease. The clinical significance of polyphonic wheezing is that it indicates widespread airways obstruction, especially if it is occurring during unforced exhalations.

Polyphonic wheezing can be generated in some normal subjects during a forced expiratory maneuver.[11] The forced expiratory wheeze results from the high flowrate of gas out of the lung through normally narrowed airways. With airways disease, the wheezing will occur at lower flowrates since the obstruction is more severe. Therefore, only wheezing heard during unforced exhalations is a reliable sign of abnormal pathology.

Paradoxical Absence of Wheezing

The absence of wheezing in a patient who previously was wheezing is consistent with severe airways obstruction that causes ventilatory failure. Rapid airflow past the site of obstruction is needed to set the airway walls in motion and create the musical sound. As the patient tires, the respiratory effort may diminish and result in less intense wheezing or no wheezing at all. This can be interpreted falsely as improvement if other clinical parameters are not assessed simultaneously. Evaluation of multiple clinical parameters such as pulse, blood pressure, and patient orientation along with the lung sounds always provides a more accurate assessment than looking at any one parameter.

Therapeutic Implications of Wheezing

Wheezing is a common clinical sign of obstructive airways disease. With obstructive defects, wheezing is often expiratory but may be heard throughout the respiratory cycle. Multiple monophonic or polyphonic wheezing is a clinical sign of widespread airways obstruction, as seen with asthma or bronchitis. In such cases, bronchodilator therapy is indicated (see Table 4-2). The intensity of the wheeze does not indicate the degree of bronchodilator response to be expected. COPD patients who wheeze are more likely to have a significant response to bronchodilators and corticosteroids than those who don't.[12]

When the wheezing varies with coughing, airway secretions may be contributing to the sound production process. Therapy to remove the excess secretions, such as aerosol treatments and postural drainage, may be indicated.

Therapy that improves the airway caliber should cause changes in the characteristics of the continuous lung sounds. As airway obstruction diminishes, the wheezing may decrease in pitch, duration and intensity. If treatment is effective, the wheezing may resolve. The absence of wheezing also can indicate ventilatory failure, as mentioned before.

Stridor

Stridor is most often an inspiratory sound that is loud and usually heard at a distance from the patient. It indicates that laryngeal or tracheal obstruction is present. Epiglottitis, viral croup, foreign body aspiration, airway inflammation following extubation, tumors and tracheal stenosis can cause stridor.

Table 4-2. Treatment Implications from Lung Sounds

Lung Sound	Possible Therapy(s)
diminished/bronchial breath sounds	lung expansion therapy postural drainage frequent turning of patient
wheezes	bronchodilators aerosol therapy
stridor	medication-nebulizer therapy aerosol/mist tent monitor patient
late-inspiratory crackles	lung expansion therapy postural drainage frequent turning of patient
coarse inspiratory and expiratory crackles	cough training suctioning hydration

Stridor is a sign of a potentially serious and life-threatening problem, especially in children. The patient with stridor must be closely watched and evaluated for signs of severe obstruction. As the obstruction worsens, stridor may become inspiratory and expiratory. The patient will begin using the accessory muscles to move air past the obstruction. Paradoxical pulse may occur. The presence of cyanosis in a patient with upper airway obstruction is a particularly ominous, troublesome sign. It indicates that airway obstruction is severe enough to cause ventilatory failure and hypoxemia.

In some cases, stridor may respond to cool mist and inhalation of racemic epinephrine. This treatment has proven beneficial in patients with airway inflammation due to laryngotracheobronchitis and following extubation. In all patients with stridor, however, close monitoring of the patient is critical and the possible need to place an artificial airway must be considered in advance.

Auscultation of the Infant

Auscultation findings in an infant are of less value than in pediatric or adult patients but are still very important. Because the infant's chest is so small, localization of the findings is difficult. Normal breath sounds in one region of the lung are transmitted easily to other areas making it difficult to identify localized areas of disease.

Normal breath sounds in neonates and pediatric patients are louder and more bronchial in character, even over peripheral regions of the chest. The degree and symmetry of air entry should be assessed bilaterally by auscultation. Diminution of air entry will be easier to identify when it is unilateral. Diminished breath sounds occur in hyaline membrane disease, atelectasis, emphysema, pneumothorax, and with shallow breathing.

Fine late-inspiratory crackles are normal findings within the first 24 hours after birth. Fine crackles are also common in pneumonia, hyaline membrane disease, and pulmonary edema. Inspiratory crackles may be identified only when the neonate takes in a deep breath which may need to be induced by stimulating a cry. Wheezes are identified with airways obstruction as when bronchiolitis or aspiration of oral feedings occurs. Auscultation over the nares may assist in the identification of grunting, an early sign of respiratory distress.

Review of Pulmonary Disorders

Atelectasis

Diffuse micro-atelectasis is common in hospitalized patients, and is related to shallow breathing. Late-inspiratory crackles over the more dependent lung zones is the usual auscultatory finding (Table 4–3). The crackles may dissipate with deep breathing maneuvers or changes in position. As the atelectasis involves more significant portions of the lung, the breath sounds may become decreased and even absent.

When entire areas of the lung collapse, (e.g., lobar atelectasis) rapid and shallow breathing is common and fever may occur. Percussion over the affected regions reveals a dull note and tactile fremitus is increased. Bronchophony, egophony, and whispered pectoriloquy may be present. If the atelectasis is not treated, pneumonia can develop.

Table 4-3. Changes in Lung Sounds with Pulmonary Disease

Lung Disease	Breath Sounds	Adventitious Lung Sound
pneumonia	bronchial or absent	inspiratory crackles
atelectasis	harsh/bronchial	late-inspiratory crackles
pneumothorax	absent	none
emphysema	diminished	early-inspiratory crackles
chronic bronchitis	normal	wheezes and crackles
pulmonary fibrosis	harsh	inspiratory crackles
congestive heart failure	diminished	inspiratory crackles
pleural effusion	diminished	none
asthma	diminished	wheezes

Pneumonia

Acute bacterial pneumonia may cause dyspnea, cough and fever. The breath sounds heard over the segments of pneumonia are determined by the degree of air entry in the affected region. If air entry is adequate, bronchial type breath sounds usually are identified. If air entry is poor, such as with mucus plugging of the airways and atelectasis, the breath sounds may be diminished or absent.

Fine late-inspiratory crackles are also common, especially in the early stages of pneumonia. Later, more coarse type crackles related to airway secretions are a frequent finding. Coughing usually causes a temporary clearing of the coarse crackles as the lung secretions are cleared.

If the pneumonic consolidation involves a sizeable area of the lung, such as with pneumonia, the percussion note over the area is dull and tactile fremitus is increased. Bronchophony, egophony, and whispered pectoriloquy are usually present. Chest expansion is reduced on the affected side.

Congestive Heart Failure

When the left ventricle fails in patients with heart disease, a build-up of fluid occurs in the lungs. The clinical findings that result depend on the degree of heart failure and fluid collection in the lungs. The patient with CHF usually complains of shortness of breath, especially at night after reclining. Initially, as fluid collects in the lungs, inspiratory crackles will be evident in the dependent regions only. As the heart failure progresses, coarse crackles will be heard, even in the non-dependent regions of the lungs.

The patient with pulmonary edema often is breathing more rapidly and with more effort than normal. Hypoxemia and its manifestations (cyanosis, tachycardia, etc.) will occur unless oxygen therapy is applied. Pink frothy sputum is often coughed up in those with acute pulmonary edema. Radiographic examination of the chest is an important evaluation tool in this disorder and correlates more closely with the severity of hemodynamic alterations than the physical examination results. With severe CHF, pleural effusions are common.

Pleural Effusion

A build-up of fluid in the pleural region will result in a significant decrease in the breath sounds. A dull percussion note will be present over the effusion. Bronchophony, egophony, and whispered pectoriloquy may be present over the upper aspect of the effusion indicative of an area of consolidated, atelectatic lung. Tactile fremitus is absent over the area covered by the effusion. If the effusion is large, the patient will be short of breath and the affected side will expand poorly. In patients with pleurisy, a friction rub commonly is heard. A friction rub is identified most easily when there is a "to-and-fro" inspiratory and expiratory coarse noise.

Pulmonary Fibrosis

Fibrosis of the alveolar and interstitial tissues of the lung results in a restrictive defect. The patient with pulmonary fibrosis often complains of dyspnea and a dry (non-productive) cough. In early stages, fine late-inspiratory crackles are heard frequently over only the dependent regions. With more advanced cases, the crackles are heard farther up the chest in the mid-lung regions. The crackles of pulmonary fibrosis are high-pitched, and have been labeled with multiple descriptive terms, e.g., velcro rales, cellophane rales, and snow-shoe rales. They do not disappear with deep breathing, coughing, or changes in position. Tachypnea, hypoxemia, and respiratory alkalosis are common.

Pneumothorax

Clinical findings are related to the extent of the pneumothorax. A small pneumothorax usually will not be identified by physical examination, it requires radiographic detection. With significant lung compression, dyspnea is likely. Breath sounds will be decreased significantly over the affected regions since sound transmits poorly through the air-filled pleural space.

A pneumothorax will result in an increase in the resonance to percussion while fremitus is decreased. Bronchophony, egophony and whispered pectoriloquy are absent. It is critical to detect a pneumothorax in a mechanically ventilated patient because a tension pneumothorax can result. In such cases, severe hypotension, reduced cardiac output and death can result, therefore, a chest tube must be put into the pleural space quickly to evacuate the air.

Asthma

When the patient with asthma is asymptomatic, breath sounds are usually normal. Mild wheezing and noisy breathing can be heard at times in between attacks. As airway obstruction ensues, the patient usually complains of dyspnea. Cough also is a frequent complaint. Expiratory wheezing is a common finding during attacks of bronchospasm. With treatment, airways obstruction may lessen; this results in less intense, shorter and/or lower pitched wheezing. If the patient tires when airway obstruction persists, wheezing also can diminish in intensity and pitch. In such cases, vital signs and peak flow assessment will demonstrate a lack of improvement in pulmonary function.

During acute episodes of asthma, the chest often hyperinflates, as a result of air trapping. Resonance to percussion is increased bilaterally and tactile fremitus is reduced mildly. The patient commonly is using the accessory respiratory muscles to breathe and appears to be working very hard to ventilate. Hypoxemia and hypercapnia can result and may increase the alteration in clinical parameters.

Chronic Bronchitis

Patients with chronic bronchitis complain of frequent coughing and sputum production. Acute episodes of airway infection can result in significant increases in airway resistance. Dyspnea and fever are common during such episodes. Auscultation commonly reveals coarse crackles, and occasionally expiratory wheezing. If the airways are free of secretions at the time of the examination, the breath sounds may be normal.

Emphysema

The patient with pulmonary emphysema typically complains of dyspnea on exertion. The breath sounds are reduced markedly bilaterally. Heart sounds are also distant due to the hyperinflation, increased anterior-posterior diameter of the chest, and large retrosternal airspace. Early inspiratory crackles may be present and a prolonged expiratory phase is common.

With emphysema, the patient usually appears to be working hard to breathe. Accessory muscle usage is common. Chest expansion is reduced bilaterally, and diaphragm movement is limited. Resonance is increased with percussion and tactile fremitus is reduced. Since it is unusual for patients with chronic obstructive pulmonary disease (COPD) to have pure emphysema or chronic bronchitis, one may find a variety of the auscultatory findings described under chronic bronchitis, emphysema, and asthma.

In early COPD, breath sounds may be normal. Timing the duration of a forced vital capacity (FVC) may be the only clue to the presence of an obstructive defect detectable by physical examination. This is accomplished by measuring how long it takes to exhale the FVC while listening over the sternum with the diaphragm of the stethoscope. Normally, one should be able to exhale the FVC within 4 seconds. With emphysema and other obstructive defects, the patient cannot exhale their FVC within 4 seconds. In fact, they may not be able to exhale their total FVC before the need to inhale overcomes their desire to continue exhaling.

References

1. Dosani, R and Kraman, SS: *Lung sound intensity variability in normal men,* Chest 83:629, 1983.

2. Bohadana, AB, Peslin, R and Uffholtz, H: *Breath sounds in the clinical assessment of airflow obstruction,* Thorax 33:345, 1978.

3. Pardee, NE, Martin, CJ and Morgan, EH: *A test of the practical value of estimating breath sound intensity,* Chest 70:341, 1976.

4. Kramin, SS: *The relationship between airflow and lung sound amplitude in normal subjects,* Chest 86:225, 1984.

5. Heckerling, PS: *The need for chest roentgenograms in adults with acute respiratory illness,* Arch Intern Med 146:1321, 1986.

6. Nath, AR and Capel, LH: *Inspiratory crackles - early and late,* Thorax 29:223, 1974.

7. Nath, AR and Capel, LH: *Lung crackles in bronchiectasis,* Thorax 35:694, 1980.

8. Thacker, RE and Kraman, SS: *The prevalence of auscultatory crackles in subjects without lung disease,* Chest 81:672, 1982.

9. Braughman, RP and Loudon, RG: *Quantification of wheezing in acute asthma,* Chest 86:718, 1984.

10. Braughman, RP and Loudon, RG: *Lung sound analysis for continuous evaluation of airflow obstruction in asthma,* Chest 88:364, 1985.

11. Husodo, HOS: *Tracheal auscultation in the differentiation of whistling sounds, heard at the chest,* Seventh International Conference on Lung Sounds, University of California, Davis School of Medicine, (Abstract, Oct. 1982).

12. Marini, JJ, Pierson, DJ, Hudson, LD and Lakshiminarayan, S: *The significance of wheezing in chronic airflow obstruction,* Am Rev Resp Dis 120:1069, 1979.

Suggested Reading

Kraman, SS: *Vesicular (normal) lung sounds: How are they made, where do they come from, and what do they mean?* Sem in Resp Med 6:183, 1985.

Polysongsang, Y: *Lung Sounds as indices of ventilation,* Sem in Resp Med 6:192, 1985.

Waring, WW; Beckerman, RC and Hopkins, RL: *Continuous adventitious lung sounds: Site and method of production and significance,* Sem in Resp Med 6:201, 1985.

Wilkins, RL: *Clinical application of lung sounds,* Current Reviews in Resp Ther 7:147, 1985.

CHAPTER 5
Case Studies

James R. Dexter
Susanne C. Lareau
Cynthia A. Cline

This chapter provides seven case studies as illustrations of how auscultation findings can be helpful especially in the assessment of patients with respiratory disease. In each case, the patient's history, physical examination findings and other clinical data are presented to provide a "clinical picture." Lung sounds for each case example have been recorded on the audio-tape and should be identified as the chest examination findings are reviewed. At the end of each case, several questions are listed to stimulate thinking. The answers to the questions are reviewed at the end of the chapter.

Case #1:

HISTORY OF PRESENT ILLNESS: A 36-year-old caucasian female with exertional dyspnea which has gradually worsened over the last several years is seen in the outpatient clinic. She had stopped jogging several years earlier because of dyspnea. She now finds that her exercise tolerance is limited to 1 block or ½ flight of stairs. The patient denies cough, sputum production, wheezing, fever, night sweats, chest pain, orthopnea or allergies. The patient knows of no aspirin sensitivity, and has no sinus congestion.

PAST MEDICAL HISTORY

Illnesses: Unknown

Familial Illnesses: Her father died of emphysema at the age of 52 and one older brother has been told he has obstructive pulmonary disease.

Occupational History: Patient has worked as a check-out clerk at a local grocery store. No exposure to known pulmonary toxins.

Pets: None

Travel: Vacation in the Southeastern United States, six months ago.

Hobbies: Fishing

Surgeries: None

Marital Status: Single

Medications: None

TB History: No exposure, no skin tests.

Smoking History: 10 pack years.

Allergies: None

PHYSICAL EXAMINATION:

General: The patient is a well nourished, well developed caucasian female in no acute distress, at rest. Affect is appropriate.

Vital Signs: Within normal limits.

HEENT: Non-contributory to the present problem.

Neck: The trachea is mid-line and mobile. There is no stridor on tidal volume or forced vital capacity maneuvers. Carotid pulsations are +2 and symmetrical and there are no carotid bruits (abnormal blood flow sounds). There is no lymphadenopathy (swelling of lymph glands). Accessory muscles are used for breathing with minimal exertion.

Chest: There is a substantially increased A-P diameter and there is decreased expansion with respiration. Increased resonance is noted upon percussion.

Heart: Cardiac sounds are mildly diminished. There is no right ventricular heave. The cardiac sounds are regular in rhythm without murmurs, gallops, or rubs.

Lungs: Refer to tape for example of lung sounds.

Abdomen: Soft and non-tender. Bowel sounds are present. The liver is percussed 2 cm below the costal margin, however the total width is only 10 cm at the midclavicular line.

Extremities: There is no cyanosis, clubbing or edema. Pulses are +2 and symmetrical in all areas.

Chest X-ray: (see Fig. 5–1)

Pulmonary Function Studies: $FEF_{25-75\%}$ is 28% of predicted. FVC is 84% of predicted, FEV_1 45% of predicted and DLCO is 48% of predicted.

QUESTIONS:
1. Describe the breath sounds heard on auscultation.
2. What pulmonary disorders can cause this patient's problem?
3. What information supports the most likely diagnosis for this patient's problems over the other possibilities?
4. What is the most likely diagnosis?
5. What physiologic principles underlie the auscultatory findings in this case?
6. Are the breath sounds consistent with the pulmonary function test results?

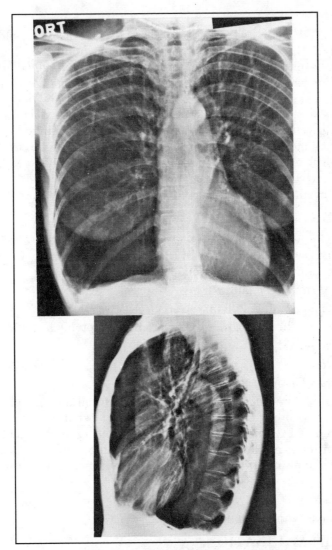

Figure 5-1   Roentgenograms of the chest in posteroanterior (A) and lateral projections (B). Both views reveal marked overinflation of the lungs with diminished vasculature in the bases and low, flat hemidiaphragms. The lateral view shows increased A-P diameter and a large retrosternal airspace.

Case #2:

HISTORY OF PRESENT ILLNESS: The patient is a 38-year-old caucasian female with a 12 month history of wheezing and gradually increasing dyspnea on exertion, despite vigorous use of a large variety of bronchodilator medications including beta agonists by both oral and inhaled routes, oral theophylline, oral and inhaled steroids, cromolyn sodium, and oral antibiotics. Other symptoms include severe morning cough and daily sputum production of approximately ¼ cup yellow to green mucous. Her cough has changed substantially over the past 6 months becoming more brassy in nature. Exercise tolerance is currently 2–3 blocks at normal pace. Patient has noticed a 5 lb. weight loss since the onset of her symptoms. Pertinent negative symptoms include the absence of chest pain, fevers, night sweats, orthopnea, and pedal edema.

PAST MEDICAL HISTORY:

Illnesses: Childhood diseases include whooping cough, measles, and mumps.

Familial Illnesses: Father had TB in 1948 and coronary artery bypass graft in 1978. Mother and 3 siblings are well.

Occupational History: Realtor

Pets: Blood hound and gold fish.

Travel: Hawaiian holiday 4 months before the symptoms began.

Hobbies: Bridge and golf.

Surgeries: None

Marital Status: Divorced for 10 years.

Medications: Metered dose inhalers (albuterol, terbutaline, beclomethasone, and cromolyn sodium), theophylline S.A. 800mg per day; oral beta agonist (metaproterenol). Prednisone (several courses of 40 mg per day each of 2 weeks duration); antibiotics: (short courses of trimethoprim/sulfamethoxazole, ampicillin, tetracycline, and erythromycin), without evidence of substantial improvement.

Smoking History: 30 pack years.

Allergies: Sensitivities to pollens and cats.

PHYSICAL EXAMINATION:

General: The patient is a well nourished, well developed caucasian female who appears slightly older than her stated age of 38. She is alert, oriented and in no acute respiratory distress sitting in a chair.

Vital Signs: Within normal limits.

HEENT: Does not provide evidence contributory to the present problem.

Neck: The trachea is midline and mobile to palpation. There is no swelling of the lymph glands (lymphadenopathy), jugular venous distention or bruits heard over the carotid arteries. Carotid pulsations are symmetrical.

CHEST: Normal A-P diameter and normal expansion with breathing.

Heart: Regular rate and rhythm without murmurs, gallops or rubs. No ventricular heaves.

Lungs: Refer to tape for example of breath sounds heard over the upper airway. Inspiratory and expiratory monophonic wheezing is heard over the upper lung fields. Faint monophonic wheezing is heard over the lower lobes.

Abdomen: Soft and non-tender to palpations. No masses or organomegally are noted. Bowel sounds are normal.

Extremities: There is no evidence of cyanosis, clubbing, or edema. Peripheral pulses are +2 and symmetrical bilaterally.

EKG: Normal

Pulmonary Function Tests: Flow volume loops show marked reduction in inspiratory flow rates. (See Fig. 5-2).

Chest X-ray: Normal

QUESTIONS:

1. Describe the breath sounds heard on auscultation over the neck.
2. What pulmonary disorders can cause this patient's problem?
3. What information supports the most likely diagnosis for this patient's problems over the other possibilities?
4. What is the most likely diagnosis?
5. What physiologic principles underlie the auscultatory findings in this case?

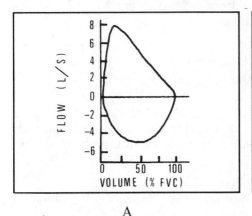 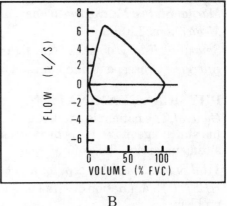

A   B

Figure 5-2   Flow volume loops showing a normal individual (A) and a patient with an extra-thoracic large airway obstruction (B). Note the plateau representing limited inspiratory flow on the inspiratory loop in figure B.

Case #3:

HISTORY OF PRESENT ILLNESS: You are requested to evaluate a 35-year-old-caucasian male who has been treated on the psychiatric ward of the hospital for approximately 30 days. He was without physical complaints until the afternoon of the request when he noticed a sharp pain in his right chest and slight dyspnea while playing ping pong. The pain was of sudden onset, got worse with breathing and improved when he held his breath. It radiated through to his back but not to his shoulder or jaw. It did not change with exercise or change in position. He has no other complaints and specifically denies a history of asthma, hay fever, and allergies. He also denies cough, fever, sputum production, night sweats, and orthopnea.

PAST MEDICAL HISTORY:

Illnesses: Childhood diseases, including measles and mumps.

Familial Illnesses: Non-contributory.

Occupational History: Truck driver for a local egg company.

Pets: Staffordshire terrier.

Travel: Patient has not been outside of Southern California.

Hobbies: Pool, ping pong and dirt bike racing.

Surgeries: Appendectomy at age 12 and tonsillectomy at age 13.

Marital Status: Married with one child.

Medications: Lithium

Smoking History: 45 pack years (started at age 12).

Allergies: Grass, penicillin, and stelazine.

PHYSICAL EXAMINATION:

General: The patient is a tall, thin caucasian male who appears approximately his stated age of 35. He is alert, oriented and in no respiratory distress while sitting up during the examination.

Vital Signs: Normal except for a pulse rate of 100.

HEENT: Examination does not provide evidence contributory to the pulmonary problem.

Neck: The trachea is mildly deviated toward the left but is mobile to palpation. There is no lymphadenopathy, jugular venous distention or carotid bruits. Carotid pulsations are +2 and symmetrical bilaterally.

Chest: The chest is asymmetrical and there is more movement on the left side with breathing. Percussion of the chest reveals increased resonance over the right chest.

Heart: Regular rate and rhythm without murmurs, gallops, or rubs. No ventricular heaves are noted.

Lungs: Refer to tape for example of lung sounds.

Abdomen: Soft and non-tender to palpation. Bowel sounds are present and no masses or organomegally are noted.

Extremities: There is no cyanosis, clubbing or edema. Pulses are +2 and symmetrical in all areas.

Chest X-ray: See Fig. 5-3.

QUESTIONS:

1. Describe the breath sounds heard on auscultation.
2. What pulmonary disorders can cause this patient's problem?
3. What information supports the most likely diagnosis for this patient's problems over the other possibilities?
4. What is the most likely diagnosis?
5. What physiologic principles underlie the auscultatory findings in this case?

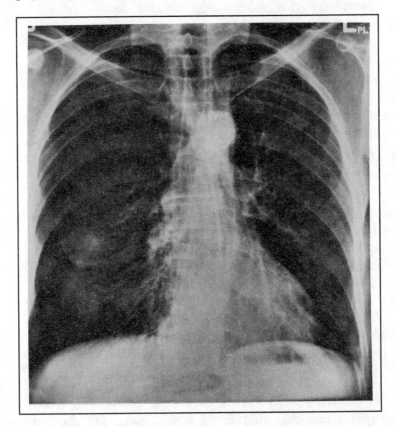

Figure 5-3 Chest roentgenogram showing partial collapse of the right lung. Note the increased density of the right lung compared to the left lung, the pleural reflection, and the leftward shift of the mediastinum.

Case #4

HISTORY OF PRESENT ILLNESS: A 40-year-old man has been cared for on the Surgery Service for approximately 5 days after a cholecystectomy. He experienced a sudden onset of dyspnea 48 hours previously while in the bathroom. The dyspnea gradually decreased in severity, however, he developed chest pain on the right side approximately 24 hours later. He denies cough, fever, night sweats, or sputum production. He denies leg tenderness or swelling and denies history of asthma, hay fever, allergies or wheezing.

PAST MEDICAL HISTORY:

Illnesses: Mild systemic hypertension.

Familial Illnesses: Father and two older brothers died of cardiac arrest.

Occupational History: The patient has worked as an auto mechanic where he was exposed to brake dust and degreasing solution fumes on a regular basis.

Pets: Goats and sheep kept in the back yard.

Travel: A recent trip to Yellowstone National Park by automobile.

Hobbies: Tending to goats and sheep.

Surgeries: Appendectomy and recent cholecystectomy.

Marital Status: Married to his third wife for 6 years.

Medications: Hydrochlorothiazide.

Smoking History: 20 pack years.

PHYSICAL EXAMINATION:

General: The patient is an obese caucasian male who appears approximately his stated age of 40. He is alert and oriented but mildly dyspneic while lying in bed during the examination.

Vital Signs: Temperature 38°C, heart rate of 98/min, respiratory rate 24/min. Blood pressure is 120/70 mmHg.

HEENT: Examination was non-contributory for the current pulmonary problem.

Neck: Trachea is mid-line and mobile to palpation, and no stridor or wheezing are noted during tidal volume breathing. Carotid pulsations were +2 and symmetrical bilaterally and there are no carotid bruits. There is no jugular venous distention or lymphadenopathy noted.

Chest: Normal AP diameter and slightly decreased expansion with respiration.

Heart: Regular rate and rhythm at approximately 98/min. apically. No murmurs, heaves, or gallops noted.

Lungs: Refer to tape for example of lung sounds.

Abdomen: Soft and non-tender to palpation. The recent surgical scar appears to be healing well and is without evidence of inflammation. Bowel sounds are present and no masses are noted. Urogenital examination was normal.

Extremities: There is no clubbing or edema. Pulses are +2 and symmetrical in all areas. There is no calf tenderness or other evidence of vein inflammation (thrombophlebitis).

Lab Work: ABG's: pH 7.48, $PaCO_2$ 30 mmHg, PaO_2 55 mmHg. CBC – WBC 15,000 mm^3, Hgb 14 gm%, Hct 47%, Segs 68%, Band 4%, Lymph 28%.

EKG: Shows slight right axis deviation.

Chest X-ray: See Fig. 5-4.

$\dot{V}/\dot{Q}$ *Lung Scan:* Demonstrates a perfusion defect in the right lower lobe with normal ventilation.

QUESTIONS:

1. Describe the breath sounds heard on auscultation.
2. What pulmonary disorders can cause this patient's problem?
3. What information supports the most likely diagnosis for this patient's problems over the other possibilities?
4. What is the most likely diagnosis?
5. What physiologic principles underlie the auscultatory findings in this case?

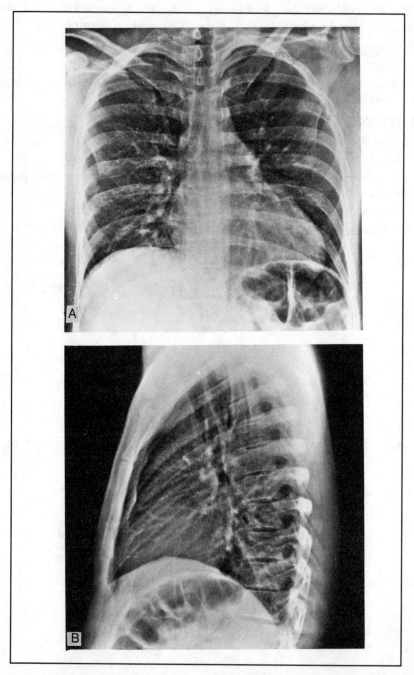

Figure 5-4 Standard P-A and lateral chest roentgenogram demonstrating increased density in the right lower lobe. The abnormality is more easily seen in the lateral projection.

Case #5

HISTORY OF PRESENT ILLNESS: The patient is a 25-year-old caucasian female school teacher who presented to the Emergency Room after a hard day of barrel racing at a local gymkhana event. She complains of severe dyspnea which began during the vigorous activity associated with her competition. She has been treated for asthma since approximately age 8 with an increasingly complex medication regimen, currently consisting of a 24 hour sustained action oral theophylline, a beta agonist metered dose inhaler used several times daily prior to exercise, and a steroid metered dose inhaler. She has not recently required oral prednisone. Her current complaints include extreme dyspnea, severe non-productive cough, a heavy sensation in her chest and a feeling of impending doom. She has taken all of her medication regularly through the day with the last dose just before her decision to visit the Emergency Room. She denies recent fever, night sweats, chills, change in sputum or peripheral edema.

PAST MEDICAL HISTORY:

Illnesses: The patient has been without medical problems except severe asthma. Broken leg at age 12 and broken arm at age 18, both from injuries sustained during horse back competition. Nasal polyps removed at age 20.

Familial Illnesses: None

Occupational History: The patient is a high school teacher.

Pets: 4 Morgan horses.

Travel: None outside California during the past 2 years.

Hobbies: Horseback competition, grooming shows.

Surgeries: None

Marital Status: Single

Medications: Oral theophylline, inhaled beta agonist, inhaled corticosteroid.

Exposures: None known.

Smoking History: None

Allergies: Dust, many pollens, aspirin, sulfa drugs and penicillin.

PHYSICAL EXAMINATION:

General: The patient is a well developed caucasian female who appears slightly younger than her stated age of 25. She is alert and oriented, but is sitting on the edge of the bed with her hands propped on her knees and is complaining of respiratory distress. She is using accessory muscles of respiration and is mildly diaphoretic (sweaty).

Vital Signs: Temperature 37°C, pulse 140/min, respirations 18/min, blood pressure 160/92 mmHg. There is a paradoxial pulse of 18 mmHg.

HEENT: Slight flaring of the nares with inspiration and cyanosis of the lips.

Neck: Full active range of motion. Trachea is mid-line and mobile to palpation and there is no stridor during tidal volume or forced vital capacity maneuvers. There is mild jugular venous distention with respiration. There is no cervical or supraclavicular lymphadenopathy. Carotid pulsations are +2 and symmetrical and there are no carotid bruits.

Chest: There is increased AP diameter and decreased expansion with respiration. The chest is moderately hyperresonant to percussion.

Heart: Regular rhythm at 140/min. There are no murmurs, gallops, or rubs. No ventricular heaves.

Lungs: Refer to tape for example of lung sounds.

Abdomen: Non-tender to palpation. The patient is not comfortable lying down so the abdominal exam was difficult to perform.

Extremities: No clubbing or edema. There was cyanosis of the nail beds on both upper and lower extermities. Pulses were +2 and symmetrical in all areas.

Pulmonary Function Test: [FEV_1 1.0 l, FVC 3.5 l]

Lab Work: ABG - pH 7.35, $PaCO_2$ 40 mmHg, PaO_2 40 mmHg. CBC - WBC = 13,000/mm^3, Hgb 13 gm%, Hct 40%, Segs 75%, Band 5%, Lymphs 20%.

Chest X-ray: See Fig. 5-5 and Fig. 5-6.

QUESTIONS:

1. Describe the breath sounds heard on auscultation.
2. What is the differential diagnosis of this patient's problem?
3. What information supports the most likely diagnosis for this patient's problems over the other possibilities.
4. What is the most likely diagnosis?
5. What physiologic principles underlie the auscultatory findings in this case? What could reduce the intensity of the sounds?

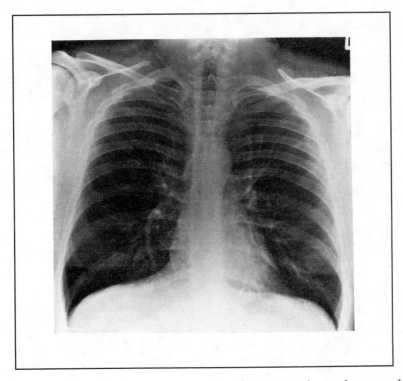

Figure 5-5 Standard P-A roentgenogram demonstrating pulmonary hyper-expansion with eleven posterior ribs visible. The cardiac silhouette and pulmonary vasculature are relatively normal in appearance. See Fig. 5-6 for the lateral projection.

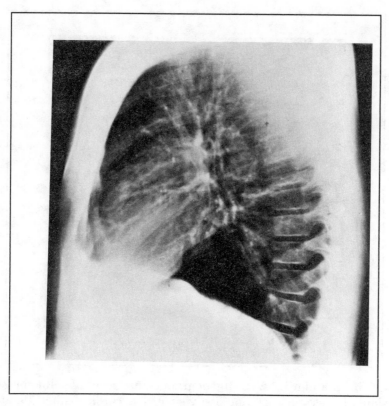

Figure 5-6   Lateral projection for the same patient as in Fig. 5-5. This view also shows pulmonary hyperexpansion with a flattened diaphragm.

Case #6

HISTORY OF PRESENT ILLNESS: The patient is a 64-year-old alcoholic male who has been admitted through the Emergency Room because of a 2 day history of cough, shaking chills, and sputum production. The sputum is yellow in color, thick and tenacious. The patient's temperature has been 39°C several times during the 2 days prior to admission. In addition to the fever, the patient complains of mild dyspnea and severe right lower chest pain during inspiration. The patient has not been eating very well and thinks he has lost about 4 pounds during the week prior to admission. He denies ankle edema, wheezing, palpations, orthopnea, or paroxysmal nocturnal dyspnea.

PAST MEDICAL HISTORY:

Illnesses: High blood pressure, mild chronic obstructive lung disease.

Familial Illnesses: None

Occupational History: Retired butcher.

Pets: None

Travel: None

Hobbies: None

Surgeries: Removal of basal cell carcinoma of his nose, sigmoid colon polypectomy, and prostatectomy.

Marital Status: Married 40 years.

Medications: Aspirin, Robitussin and Sudafed.

Smoking History: 40 pack years.

Allergies: Sinequan and thorazine.

PHYSICAL EXAMINATION:

General: Thin, caucasian male in mild respiratory distress at rest in the hospital bed. He complains primarily of pain in his right chest with respiration. His intellect is nearly normal, his affect is anxious.

Vital Signs: Temperature 38.5°C, pulse 110/min., respirations 28/min., blood pressure 150/94 mmHg.

HEENT: Exam was found to be non-contributory to the present problem.

Neck: Supple with full active range of motion. Trachea mid-line and mobile to palpation. No stridor is noted during either tidal volume or forced vital capacity maneuvers. Carotid pulsations are +2 and symmetrical and there are no carotid bruits. There is no cervical or supraclavicular lymphadenopathy. There is no jugular venous distention.

Chest: Normal antero-posterior diameter, but slightly decreased expansion with respiration, particularly on the right side. There is normal resonance to percussion over most of the chest except the right lower chest which has decreased resonance.

Heart: Regular rate and rhythm. There are no murmurs, gallops or rubs and no heaves.

Lungs: Refer to tape for example of lung sounds.

Abdomen: Soft and non-tender to palpation. Bowel sounds are present and the liver is of normal span in the mid-clavicular line. No masses are noted.

Extremities: There is no cyanosis, clubbing, or edema. Pulses are +2 and symmetrical in all areas.

Lab Work: CBC - WBC 24,000/mm^3, Hgb 11 gm%, Hct 40%, Segs 80%, Bands 15%, Lymphs 5%.

Chest Film: See Fig. 5-7.

QUESTIONS:

1. Describe the breath sounds heard on auscultation.
2. What pulmonary disorders can cause this patient's problem?
3. What information supports the most likely diagnosis for this patient's problems over the other possibilities?
4. What is the most likely diagnosis?
5. What physiologic principles underlie the auscultatory findings in this case?

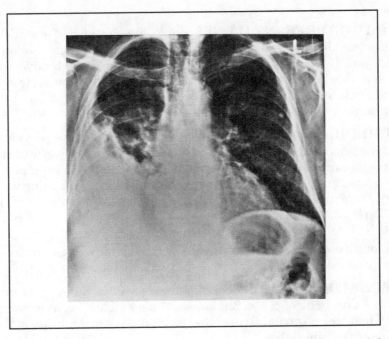

Figure 5-7 Chest roentgenogram demonstrating consolidation of the right lower lobe.

Case #7:

HISTORY OF PRESENT ILLNESS: A 28-week estimated gestational age male neonate diagnosed with Respiratory Distress Syndrome, is on a 45% oxygen hood. He has had increasing episodes of apnea and bradycardia. His respiratory rate has increased from 50 to 80 in the last few hours. He is having moderate substernal and intercostal retractions. The patient has a normal temperature.

PAST MEDICAL HISTORY: The patient was born 5 days previously to a 17-year-old gravida 2 para 1 AbO caucasion female with a history of smoking during pregnancy. Delivery was normal with a spontaneous vaginal delivery. Apgars were 2 and 6. Resuscitation included intubation and bagging with 100% oxygen. The patient was placed on mechanical ventilation with FIO_2's greater than 60% for 4 days. Chest x-ray revealed a ground glass appearance consistent with RDS.

On the fourth day of life, the patient showed rapid improvement in blood gases and was weaned from the ventilator, extubated and placed on oxygen by hood.

MATERNAL HISTORY: Mother claims no previous illnesses or surgeries. She denies drug or alcohol use. She smoked 1 pack cigarettes/day during pregnancy. There was no prenatal care other than one visit to the doctor at 26 weeks gestation for possible labor.

This pregnancy was uneventful except for the onset of premature labor at 28 weeks.

PHYSICAL EXAMINATION

General: The patient is a 6-day-old premature male neonate who appears to be in moderate respiratory distress. He appears to be active and alert. His color appears pale on the trunk and extremities.

Vital Signs: Weight 1200 grams, heart rate 180/min., respiratory rate 80/min., temperature 37.2°C, blood pressure 60/30 mmHg.

HEENT: Non-contributory to the present problem.

Neck: The trachea is midline and mobile in palpation. Carotid pulsations are symmetrical.

Heart: Regular rate and rhythm without murmurs, gallops or rubs.

Lungs: Refer to tape for example of lung sounds.

Chest: The chest is symmetrical with equal expansion during respiration. Moderate intercostal and substernal retractions are noted. The precordium is hyperdynamic.

Extremities: There is no cyanosis or edema. Pulses are bounding and symmetrical.

CXR: Increased pulmonary vascularity, mild cardiomegaly. The lung parenchyma appears normal.

Lab Work: ABG's - pH 7.26, $PaCO_2$ 50 mmHg, PaO_2 46 mmHg. CBC - within normal limits.

QUESTIONS:
1. Describe the breath sounds heard on auscultation.
2. What is the differential diagnosis of the patient's problem?
3. What information supports the most likely diagnosis for this patient's problems over the other possibilities.
4. What is the most likely diagnosis?
5. What physiologic principles underlie the auscultatory findings in this case.

Answers to Questions for Case Examples

Answers and Discussion for Case #1:

Purpose of Case: Differentiate asthma vs. emphysema based on loudness of breath sounds and other findings.

Diagnosis: Emphysema secondary to alpha$_1$ antitrypsin deficiency.

1. Describe the breath sounds heard on auscultation.

    Breath sounds are very quiet in all lung fields and there is no evidence of stridor, wheezing or crackles.

2. What pulmonary disorders can cause this patient's problem?

    Asthma, cystic fibrosis, and emphysema.

3. What information supports the most likely diagnosis for this patient's problems over the other possibilities?

    The patient's diminished breath sounds with no crackles or wheezes during normal respiration are evidence against asthma and cystic fibrosis. Her physical exam and chest x-ray reveal pulmonary hyperexpansion and the patient's familial history of obstructive lung disease increases the likelihood of a hereditary abnormality.

4. What is the most likely diagnosis?

    Emphysema due to alpha$_1$ antitrypsin deficiency.

5. What physiologic principles underlie the auscultatory findings in this case?

    This patient with alpha$_1$ antitrypsin deficiency has lost elastic recoil in her lung, therefore distal bronchioles collapse during early expiration and the lung becomes hyperexpanded. This severely limits expiratory airflow throughout the bronchial tree and prevents the development of turbulence. Hyperexpanded lung fields transmit sounds poorly. The result is diminished lung and heart sounds.

6. Are the breath sounds consistent with the PFT results?

    Yes, the PFT results demonstrate obstructive lung disease that results in pulmonary hyperinflation and reduced transmission of breath sounds to the chest wall.

Answers and Discussion for Case #2:

Purpose of Case: Differentiate lower from upper airway obstruction based on type of wheeze and radiation.

Diagnosis: Laryngeal carcinoma.

1. Describe the breath sounds heard on auscultation over the neck.

    At the neck there is stridor present during inspiration and expiration.

2. What pulmonary disorders can cause this patient's problem?

Epiglottitis, asthma, and partial upper airway obstruction.

3. What information supports the most likely diagnosis for this patient's problems over the other possibilities?

The lack of response to bronchodilators, the brassy progressive cough, the monophonic nature of the wheeze, the uniform distribution of the wheeze heard best over upper airway and gradually diminishing in intensity toward the bases make this more likely a single source wheeze than the multiple notes that would be expected to occur in asthma with many small airways vibrating. Symptoms of epiglottitis would be of acute onset.

4. What is the most likely diagnosis?

Partial upper airway obstruction.

5. What physiologic principles underlie the auscultatory findings in this case?

Wheezing and stridor are produced by vibration of the airway wall. The pitch of the sound is determined by the characteristics of the vibrating wall of the airway and is independent of the diameter or length of the airway in which the vibrations occur. Because mass and elasticity of the bronchial wall determine the note produced when it vibrates, a disease affecting many bronchi of varying sizes would produce a polyphonic wheeze as opposed to a disease affecting only one bronchus, the larynx or the trachea. The wheeze or stridor of upper airway obstruction is more prominent during inspiration in many cases because it is extrathoracic in origin and is loudest over the neck. (See Chapter 3).

Answers and Discussion for Case #3:

Purpose of Case: Demonstrate abnormalities associated with pneumothorax.

Diagnosis: Pneumothorax on right side.

1. Describe the breath sounds heard on auscultation.

There are diminished breath sounds on the right side and normal breath sounds on the left side of the chest. Percussion reveals increased resonance on the right side. There are no wheezes or crackles.

2. What pulmonary disorders can cause this patient's problem?

Spontaneous pneumothorax, aspirated foreign body, pneumonia or pulmonary embolus.

3. What information supports the most likely diagnosis for this patient's problems over the other possibilities?

The sudden onset of chest pain and dyspnea points to an acute event. The asymmetrical chest with diminished respiratory excursions on the right side would be consistent with the pneumothorax. Increased resonance to percussion on the right side is compatible with excess air in the right thoracic cavity.

Decreased breath sounds on the larger side indicates either absence of airflow in that bronchial tree or acoustical dampening between the bronchial tree and the chest wall or both.

4. What is the most likely diagnosis?

Spontaneous right pneumothorax.

5. What physiologic principles underlie the auscultatory findings in this case?

The elastic recoil of the lung normally counterbalances the tendency of the ribs to expand. When a pneumothorax occurs, the pulmonary elastic recoil is lost and the chest wall expands unopposed. If a substantial amount of air leaks out of the lung and accumulates in the thoracic space, the mediastinal structures can be pushed toward the other side (tension pneumothorax) causing the trachea to deviate towards the opposite side away from the pneumothorax. The absence of lung expansion with respiration on the side of the pneumothorax would decrease sound generation on that side and the large accumulation of air within the pleural space would dampen breath sounds generated in the trachea and mainstem bronchus.

Answers and Discussion for Case #4:

Purpose of Case: Demonstrate pleural friction rub.
Diagnosis: Pulmonary Embolus.

1. Describe the breath sounds heard on auscultation.

Normal breath sounds with an inspiratory and expiratory pleural friction rub.

2. What pulmonary disorders can cause this patient's problem?

Pneumonia or pulmonary embolus.

3. What information supports the most likely diagnosis for this patient's problems over the other possibilities?

The predisposing factors, surgery and bed rest, associated with the sudden onset of dyspnea during exercise. The evidence for pulmonary embolus is strengthened by the pleural friction rub although that could also occur with pneumonia. The ABG showing hypocapnia and hypoxemia, fever, and leukocytosis can all be seen with both pulmonary embolus and pneumonia. A $\dot{V}/\dot{Q}$ lung scan was needed to confirm the diagnosis of pulmonary embolism. With pneumonia, both ventilation and perfusion are generally impaired.

4. What is the most likely diagnosis?

Pulmonary embolus.

5. What physiologic principles underlie the auscultatory findings in this case?

The affected pleural surface becomes inflamed. It no longer slides freely over the parietal pleura but rather moves in small increments producing many discrete discontinuous sounds or crackles much like the bow of a violin against the strings.

Answers and Discussion for Case #5:

Purpose of Case: Demonstrate wheezing during severe bronchospasm.

Diagnosis: Severe asthma.

1. Describe the breath sounds heard on auscultation.

   There is severe expiratory wheezing noted.

2. What pulmonary disorders can cause this patient's problem?

   Exacerbation of the patient's asthma, pulmonary embolus, pneumonia or bronchitis.

3. What information supports the most likely diagnosis for this patient's problems over the other possibilities?

   The history of asthma requiring multiple daily medications with a rather sudden onset of worsening during an activity associated with exposure to dust and animal dander.

4. What is the most likely diagnosis?

   Status asthmaticus.

5. What physiologic principles underlie the auscultatory findings in this case? What could reduce the intensity of the sounds?

   Production of wheezing is dependent upon bronchial wall vibration which is produced by rapid airflow through a partially obstructed airway. In this case, the patient is still able to generate sufficient airflow to produce loud wheezing. When airflow within the bronchus is sufficiently diminished, it no longer affects the bronchial wall enough to cause vibration, and wheezing diminishes. With extreme airway obstruction, airflow may be so impaired that wheezing disappears. Bronchodilitation also could result in reduced intensity of the wheezing. Careful assessment of numerous parameters is needed to interpret the changes in lung sounds.

Answers and Discussion for Case #6:

Purpose of Case: Demonstrate lung sound changes associated with lobar consolidation.

Diagnosis: Lobar pneumonia in right lower lobe.

1. Describe the breath sounds heard on auscultation.

   There are tracheobronchial breath sounds with egophony limited to the right posterior lower chest.

2. What pulmonary disorders can cause this patient's problem?

   Pneumonia, bronchogenic carcinoma, and pulmonary embolus.

3. What information supports the most likely diagnosis for this patient's problems over the other possibilities?

The clinical history of fever, chills, sputum production, dyspnea and chest pain in an alchoholic are most consistent with pneumonia. The breath sounds reveal the typical findings associated with lung consolidation, including bronchial breathing and egophony. Chest x-ray confirms the presence of a lobar pneumonia.

4. What is the most likely diagnosis?

Pneumonia (sputum culture grew Streptococcus pneumoniae).

5. What physiologic principles underlie the auscultatory findings in this case?

Sound is transmitted readily through the airways. The frequencies above 200 HTZ are filtered by normal lung tissue at a rate of 15 decibels per octave. Breath sounds are dependent upon turbulence in the large airways and are predominantly a high frequency sound. Spoken sounds are also high frequency. Lung consolidation provides a direct path for sound transmission from the larger airways to the chest wall. This allows turbulent airflow sounds in the bronchus, whispered sounds and spoken sounds to be transmitted to the chest wall with more intensity and clarity.

Answers and Discussion for Case #7

Purpose of Case: Demonstrate pulmonary edema associated with patent ductus arteriosus.

Diagnosis: Left to right shunting through a patent ductus arteriosus.

1. Describe the breath sounds heard on auscultation.

Medium inspiratory and expiratory crackles.

2. What is the differential diagnosis of this patient's problem?

Pneumonia, pulmonary edema, bronchopulmonary dysplasia (BPD).

3. What information supports the most likely diagnosis for this patient's problems over the other possibilities.

Crackles in the neonate usually indicate excess fluid in the lungs (pulmonary edema, pneumonia). The breath sounds in BPD are usually wheezing or diminished breath sounds. Increased episodes of apnea and bradycardia are associated with both patent ductus arteriosis (PDA) and pneumonia. The presence of a hyperdynamic precordium, bounding pulses and suspected pulmonary edema are all indications of a left to right shunt through the ductus arteriosus causing capillary congestion and pulmonary edema. Blood gases indicate a combined respiratory and metabolic acidosis, possibly due to decreased perfusion of the post-ductal organs. The normal CBC and stable temperature may support the diagnosis of pulmonary edema over pneumonia. The chest x-ray shows no infiltrates or changes consistent with BPD.

4. What is the most likely diagnosis?

   Pulmonary edema caused by left to right shunt through the PDA.

5. What physiologic principles underlie the auscultatory findings in this case?

   The crackles are produced when there is movement of air through secretions or fluid in the lungs, and from atelectatic small airways popping open.

A P P E N D I X   A

EXAMPLES OF LUNG SOUNDS ON AUDIO-TAPE

Adult Lung Sounds

1. Tracheobronchial breath sounds
2. Bronchovesicular breath sounds
3. Vesicular breath sounds
4. Diminished breath sounds
5. Abnormal tracheobronchial or tubular breath sounds heard over lung consolidation*
6. Fine inspiratory crackles
7. Medium inspiratory and expiratory crackles
8. Coarse inspiratory and expiratory crackles
9. Fine, late-inspiratory crackles typical for pulmonary fibrosis
10. Mild expiratory wheeze
11. Medium inspiratory crackles with moderate expiratory wheezes
12. Medium inspiratory crackles with severe expiratory wheezes
13. Pleural friction rub (heard on inspiration and expiration)
14. Inspiratory and expiratory stridor
15. Bone crepitus
16. Subcutaneous emphysema
17. Chest hair rubbing against the diaphragm of the stethoscope
18. Normal voice sounds followed by egophony
19. Normal voice sounds followed by bronchophony
20. Normal whispered sound followed by whispered pectoriloquy

Infant Lung Sounds

21. Tracheobronchial breath sounds
22. Vesicular breath sounds
23. Vesicular breath sounds with crying
24. Stridor
25. Fine inspiratory crackles
26. Medium inspiratory and expiratory crackles
27. Expiratory grunting
28. Inspiratory and expiratory low-pitched wheezes
29. Water in tubing with patient on CPAP system

*Courtesy of Dr. Roy Donnerberg

APPENDIX B

POST-TEST*

1. Airflow through which airways is normally more rapid and turbulent?
   A. trachea and main stem bronchi
   B. lobar bronchi
   C. segmental bronchi
   D. terminal bronchioles

2. Which lobes dominate the surface area of the posterior chest wall?
   A. lower lobes
   B. middle lobes
   C. upper lobes
   D. none of the above

3. The term infant's lung has approximately how many alveoli?
   A. 10 million
   B. 25 million
   C. 55 million
   D. 100 million

4. A chronic productive cough that is worse in the morning is a frequent finding in patients with:
   A. asthma
   B. chronic bronchitis
   C. emphysema
   D. pneumonia

5. Which of the following can cause the patient to feel short of breath?
   A. increased airways resistance
   B. decreased lung compliance
   C. decreased chest wall compliance
   D. all the above

6. Characteristics of pleuritic chest pain includes all of the following except:
   A. predominately present during exhalation
   B. sharp
   C. located laterally
   D. may be reduced by splinting

*For individuals interested in obtaining continuing education credit, please write: Department of Respiratory Therapy, Nichol Hall, Room 1926, Loma Linda University, Loma Linda, CA 92350

7. Which of the following are correct statements with regards to the technique for auscultation of lung sounds?
   A. begin with the lower lobes
   B. ask patient to breathe a little deeper than normal
   C. use the diaphragm piece
   D. all the above

8. Tactile fremitus is increased with:
   A. lung consolidation
   B. emphysema
   C. pleural effusion
   D. pneumothorax

9. Paradoxical pulse is a common finding in patients with:
   A. pneumonia
   B. severe airways obstruction
   C. pneumothorax
   D. chronic bronchitis

10. Decreased resonance during chest percussion is found in patients with:
    A. pneumonia
    B. pneumothorax
    C. emphysema
    D. chronic bronchitis

11. Which of the following breath sounds normally has a pause between the inspiratory and expiratory components?
    A. tracheal
    B. bronchial
    C. bronchovesicular
    D. vesicular

12. Which of the following often causes the breath sounds to become more bronchial (tubular) over the peripheral chest?
    A. emphysema
    B. pneumothorax
    C. asthma
    D. pneumonia

13. Which of the following typically causes late-inspiratory crackles to be identi-fied during auscultation?
    A. asthma
    B. pulmonary fibrosis
    C. emphysema
    D. pneumothorax

14. Which of the following qualifying adjectives has no logical basis and probably should not be used?
   A. dry
   B. fine
   C. high-pitched
   D. early inspiratory

15. Discontinuous adventitious lung sounds are best described as:
   A. wheezes
   B. crackles
   C. rales
   D. rhonchi

16. Which of the following often causes a bilateral reduction in breath sound intensity?
   A. emphysema
   B. pneumonia
   C. pulmonary edema
   D. pulmonary fibrosis

17. A major part of the confusion regarding the terminology for lung sounds has centered around use of the term:
   A. rales
   B. crackles
   C. rhonchi
   D. stridor

18. An increase in vocal resonance (bronchophony) is heard over the chest of patients with:
   A. emphysema
   B. pneumothorax
   C. chronic bronchitis
   D. pneumonia

19. Fine-inspiratory crackles in the neonate are found in:
   A. the first 24 hours of life
   B. hyaline membrane disease
   C. pulmonary edema
   D. all the above

20. What therapy is often needed to treat a patient with late-inspiratory crackles?
   A. bronchodilators
   B. artificial airway
   C. lung expansion therapy
   D. antibiotics

21. As airways obstruction decreases, the patient's wheezes may decrease in:
    A. pitch
    B. intensity
    C. duration
    D. all the above

22. Which of the following adventitious sounds is typical for patients with laryngeal or tracheal obstruction?
    A. rales
    B. crackles
    C. expiratory wheezes
    D. stridor

23. Coarse inspiratory and expiratory crackles are consistent with:
    A. pneumothorax
    B. excessive airway secretions
    C. emphysema
    D. pleural effusion

24. Diminished breath sounds in the neonate occur in:
    A. hyaline membrane disease
    B. pneumothorax
    C. atelectasis
    D. all the above

25. Clinical findings typical for pulmonary fibrosis include all the following except:
    A. fine inspiratory crackles
    B. dry cough
    C. dyspnea
    D. decreased tactile fremitus

SUBJECT INDEX